Worship in a Time of Pandemic: Fresh Possibilities and Troubling Inequalities

Worship in a Time of Pandemic: Fresh Possibilities and Troubling Inequalities

Guest Editor

Edward Foley

MDPI

Basel • Beijing • Wuhan • Barcelona • Belgrade • Novi Sad • Cluj • Manchester

Guest Editor
Edward Foley
Word and Worship
Catholic Theological Union
Chicago
USA

Editorial Office
MDPI AG
Grosspeteranlage 5
4052 Basel, Switzerland

This is a reprint of the Special Issue, published open access by the journal *Religions* (ISSN 2077-1444), freely accessible at: https://www.mdpi.com/journal/religions/special_issues/worship_pandemic.

For citation purposes, cite each article independently as indicated on the article page online and as indicated below:

Lastname, Firstname, Firstname Lastname, and Firstname Lastname. Article Title. *Journal Name* **Year**, *Volume Number*, Page Range.

ISBN 978-3-7258-5857-6 (Hbk)
ISBN 978-3-7258-5858-3 (PDF)
https://doi.org/10.3390/books978-3-7258-5858-3

Contents

About the Editor

Edward Foley

Edward Foley is the Duns Scotus Professor Emeritus of Spirituality at the Catholic Theological Union. As a self-identified practical theologian and active Roman Catholic priest, Foley's work ranges across topics in the fields of liturgy, preaching, music, religion and science, and the arts. A prolific author of over 30 books and dozens of peer review articles, his work has been translated into nine languages. The recipient of national and international awards, he is also the recipient of major grants from the John Templeton and the Lilly Endowment in preaching, science, and neuroscience.

Preface

The global pandemic of 2020 triggered drastic changes in the practices of worship for a multiplicity of believers across the religious landscape. Surprisingly to some, many of those changes are still with us years later.

On the one hand, the multiplicity of digital responses to COVID-19 provided access for millions of people to participate in worship beyond geographic, and even religious, boundaries. On the other hand, such forays into technology excluded many without digital access to live-streamed worship, highlighting existing inequities in worship and society. This Reprint examines the upheaval in worship practices sparked by the pandemic, as well as the theology around these evolving practices.

Based on the presupposition that worship itself is to be a just act, authors give special attention to the ethical implications of these emerging liturgical practices in pondering how liturgy and the allied field of liturgical studies might contribute to distributive, racial, gender, and other forms of justice. In the process, this Reprint contributes to the need for ongoing theologizing in a world of increasing liquidity, and the parallel ritual liquidity that marks 21st century worship.

Edward Foley
Guest Editor

religions

MDPI

Article

Time for Solidarity: Liturgical Time in Disaster Capitalism

Mark Roosien

Institute of Sacred Music, Yale University, New Haven, CT 06511, USA; mark.roosien@yale.edu

Abstract: This article identifies the upheaval of many people's experience of time during the COVID-19 pandemic as part of a larger phenomenon of the 24/7 temporality that can be seen to contribute to the environmental destruction and social fragmentation typical of disaster capitalism. It then proposes liturgical temporality as an alternative to 24/7 temporality, framing it as a fitting context for the cultivation of solidarity between human beings and between human beings and the natural world. It argues that modern Jewish and Christian theologies of Sabbath-keeping as a mode of liturgical and ethical praxis have articulated a liberative vision for shared liturgical temporality but have not paid sufficient attention to concrete, collective modes of liturgical time keeping that could contend with the all-encompassing reality of 24/7 life. It concludes by discussing three ways that a more robust spirituality and praxis of liturgical time could support the cultivation of solidarity: a sense of the present that is mindful of the past and future, the invitation of practitioners into a shared story, and meaningful repetition toward the appropriation of a vision of redemption and liberation for human and non-human life.

Keywords: liturgy; worship; pandemic; time; capitalism; ritual; liberation theology; Sabbath; COVID-19; ethics

1. Introduction

The COVID-19 pandemic altered the everyday experience of time for many people living in modernized, Western societies. As in-person social gatherings were largely replaced by virtual ones, the boundaries between home and work, rest and waking, and personal time and professional time significantly eroded. The pandemic seemed to create a protracted liminal time: a period of uncertainty after previous structures of life had been upended, but new, stable structures had yet to form (see Bell 2021). However, pandemic time was not so much an interruption of a previous, "normal" time as it was an acceleration of what media theorist Jonathan Crary has called the 24/7 time of late capitalism, a temporal regime in which market forces seek to extract maximum profit value from each moment, whether one is on or off the clock (Crary 2013). The rise of 24/7 time in the last two decades has been aided by the growing ubiquity of smart technologies that allow for productivity and consumption to proceed without pause for shared breaks or vacations. Accelerated during the COVID-19 pandemic, 24/7 time is a new *temporality* for the twenty-first century: a horizon of meaning by which and through which individuals experience the temporal dimension of life.

Critics argue that 24/7 temporality—time as digitalized, monetized, and relentlessly ongoing—is catastrophically unsuited for human and non-human flourishing. It enables environmental destruction, economic inequality, and social fragmentation (Chan 2020, p. 2). As media theorist Nadine Chan has recently written, the individualized digital life-worlds of 24/7 temporality take us "further away from contemporaneous and inhabited ecological time." (Chan 2020, p. 2). Those concerned with the short- and long-term perils of capitalist temporality have long sought strategies to transcend or resist this temporal regime.[1] Yet 24/7 time presents a new challenge since individual efforts to imagine new temporalities become easily trapped in the very fragmented, asynchronous lifeworlds that

24/7 time creates. How might people, in Chan's words, "learn to be contemporaneous together" under the 24/7 regime? (Chan 2020, p. 6).

In this paper, I propose that liturgical temporality could provide an alternative temporal context for religious communities to cultivate solidarity in all its dimensions: economic, social, ecological, and spiritual.[2] During the COVID-19 pandemic, religious communities struggled to maintain connection with their liturgical rhythms. Yet this struggle, too, was not new to the pandemic; it merely revealed with stark clarity the fundamental discordance between liturgical temporality and late capitalist temporality. In recent decades, Christian and Jewish theologians have noted this discordance and explored Sabbath-keeping as means of resisting inhumane time cycles. Modern theologians of Sabbath-keeping provide a useful framework for imagining shared liturgical time as a context for liberative practices of rest, prayer, gathering, protest, and critique. However, most do not offer concrete strategies for living in liturgical temporality in ways that could challenge the all-encompassing reality of 24/7 life. A more robust articulation of liturgical temporality that builds upon Sabbath practices and spiritualities but more fully embraces daily, weekly, seasonal, and annual aspects of time could provide a stronger framework for communities to practice what Pope Francis calls "habits of solidarity." Such habits can inspire people to adopt a "new mindset which thinks in terms of community and the priority of the life of all over the appropriation of goods by a few." (Francis 2013, para. 188). Additionally, "when they are put into practice, [they] open the way to other structural transformations and make them possible." (Francis 2013, para. 189). Drawing from philosopher Christina Gschwandtner's recent phenomenological study of Orthodox Christian liturgical temporality, I narrate specific ways that it could serve as a shared spiritual and practical horizon in which to cultivate solidarity between people of various groups and between human beings and the earth, and offer an alternative to the present temporal order of consumption, waste, and the reckless pursuit of profit.

2. 24/7: The Temporality of Disaster Capitalism

During the pandemic, it was often difficult to determine what day it was, an experience social media users wryly dubbed "Blursday."[3] For many, the experience of time was filtered through digital media that operated on 24/7 timeframes: virtual classrooms, social media, Zoom and other video conferencing software, video streaming and retail sites, etc.[4] Lockdowns forced many to dwell almost continuously within digital spaces, which in turn allowed the pace of consumption to proceed uninhibited by the restrictions of shared periods of rest or vacation. As a result, large tech and retail corporations, such as Amazon and Google, posted record-breaking profit numbers in 2020.[5] Measures taken out of necessity during the pandemic, such as working from home, will likely remain in place after the pandemic is over and further perpetuate the erasure of boundaries between work and home, and on-the-clock and off-the-clock time.[6] The success of corporate conglomerates and the upward transfer of wealth during the pandemic vindicates the "disaster capitalism" thesis that large corporations and wealthy individuals often benefit from social and environmental upheaval.[7] In this way, the COVID-19 pandemic was a moment of truth that accelerated the rise of 24/7 temporality already underway. It also revealed the extent to which those at the top of social and economic hierarchies benefit from this temporal regime to the detriment of other human beings and the earth. Disaster capitalism and disaster temporality come as a pair, leaving environmental destruction and social fragmentation in their wake.[8]

The record corporate profits generated under pandemic conditions represent only the most recent example of how market forces organize time in ways that maximize monetary yield.[9] More than half century ago, historian Jacques Le Goff made the influential argument that, beginning in the high middle ages, "merchant's time", measured by fixed calculations of minutes and hours, gradually displaced Western Europe's looser, shared rhythms of "church's time." The latter was determined by the liturgical offices and seasons of the church, measured by sundials and crude water clocks, and announced by bells. Merchant's time inaugurated the extractive attitude toward time neatly encapsulated in the phrase "time is money" and was (at first) vehemently attacked by the church. [10] Crary argues that twenty-first-century 24/7 temporality not only perpetuates this extractive attitude toward time but also constitutes a genuinely new horizon for temporal experience. Crary writes that 24/7 temporality, "can be characterized as a generalized inscription of human life into duration *without breaks*, defined by a principle of continuous functioning. It is a time that no longer passes, beyond clock time." (Crary 2013, p. 8). In 24/7 temporality, all days become Blursday.[11]

24/7 temporality is not simply a continuous capture of one's attention but is also a dense layering of time in which multiple things (ads, clicks, Tweets) embedded in a single visual/temporal space can be attended to in a nearly simultaneous instant. Smart technologies have created new rhythms, speeds, and formats through which actions can be easily monetized, even actions as subtle as resting one's gaze momentarily upon an image on the screen of a smartphone (Crary 2013, p. 39). Time is experienced as a constantly reloading "now" that seems ever new. However, despite their differing content, digital experiences are created to be interchangeable and thus monetizable. Global markets rely on the predictable actions of large populations and benefit from the sameness and repetition at work in digital lifeworlds (Crary 2013, p. 56). The paradoxically repetitive newness of digitally-mediated human interaction with the world, Crary argues, encourages practices that are indifferent to past or future horizons—except, perhaps, a short-term future dominated by desire for all-too-finite satisfactions.[12] One might hold onto the false hope that one more click will open up something genuinely new to counter the monotony in which one is immersed, but it is not meant to be (Crary 2013, p. 88).

The widespread habitation of digital lifeworlds with their own disjunctive temporalities would seem to preclude the formation of a shared temporality capable of contending with 24/7 time. However, Nadine Chan saw a flicker of hope for asynchronous solidarity during the COVID-19 pandemic. She argues that the social lockdowns necessitated by the two-week incubation period of the coronavirus created the possibility of a "collective, explosive, revolutionary time." Such a collective, revolutionary time was witnessed in the summer 2020 Black Lives Matter resurgence in the U.S. and around the world as people gathered together in streets and plazas, often at unpredictable times, to protest racial oppression (Chan 2020, p. 6). Chan writes, "Amid the energies of collective action, digital *asynchrony* may also be the path towards inhabited futures that are not so [digital]."[13] Chan is cautiously optimistic that a reimagination of a shared, collective future could take place amidst the proliferation of digital temporalities, a future in which multiple groups and individuals could act in solidarity to resist to the destructive practices and demands of disaster capitalism.

While digital technology is certain to be part of any future temporal arrangement, it is uncertain that the present fragmented, asynchronous temporality of 24/7 life can allow for a sustainable maintenance of solidarity. Crary holds that digital lifeworlds are ineffective as contexts for collective action since "overlaid onto them are all the *practices of individual time management* made possible by 24/7 networks and markets."[14] While digital lifeworlds provide a platform for inspired creativity and expression, their temporal frame remains firmly rooted in timekeeping habits designed to be monetized, exploited, and individualized. Indeed, because of the market's demand for homogeneity and substitutability, Crary contends that 24/7 temporality is incompatible with "any social behaviors that have a rhythmic pattern of action and pause. This would include any social exchange involving sharing, reciprocity or cooperation." (Crary 2013, p. 125). Solidarity is hence likely to be most sustainable when it is rooted in *shared* temporality, which seems elusive within the 24/7 time of disaster capitalism.[15]

3. Sabbath as Resistance to 24/7 Temporality: Promise and Pitfalls

What are the possibilities for forming a shared temporality? Recently, both religious and non-religious people alike have sought out timekeeping practices as seemingly mundane as napping and doing nothing (intentionally) through which to transcend or resist 24/7 time.[16] Since the mid-twentieth century, Jewish and Christian theologians have framed the keeping of the Sabbath as an antidote to the frantic speed of modern life. The accounts of these theologians are worth exploring as a point of departure for religious communities seeking a liberative spirituality in which to "be contemporaneous together" in solidarity. However, they often fall short of meaningfully contending with the all-encompassing nature of 24/7 temporality, both by neglecting to recommend concrete shared practices of timekeeping and overlooking the crucial role of capitalist ideology as the source of the temporality they oppose.

The most important theological consideration of the Sabbath in the twentieth century is arguably the classic 1951 book by American–Polish rabbi and philosopher Abraham Joshua Heschel, *The Sabbath: Its Meaning for Modern Man* (1951). Heschel frames Sabbath keeping as an important spiritual and social practice for Jews in the twentieth century. He writes, "Is our civilization a way to disaster, as many of us are prone to believe? . . . The faith of the Jew is not a way out of this world, but a way of being within and above this world; not to reject but to surpass civilization. The Sabbath is the day on which we learn the art of *surpassing* civilization." (Heschel 1951, p. 26). In Heschel's view, the Sabbath is a way of keeping time that allows individuals and communities to transcend the anxiety-inducing temporality of modern life while remaining active participants in society and working for its improvement.[17]

Many Christian theologians have drawn from Heschel's social–spiritual account of the Sabbath. In her 1989 book, *Keeping the Sabbath Wholly: Ceasing, Resting, Embracing, Feasting*, Christian theologian Marva J. Dawn cites the Sabbath practice of rest from work on Sunday or Saturday to inform broader practices of "ceasing, resting, embracing, [and] feasting," as per the subtitle of the book.[18] Pope John Paul II, in his 1998 apostolic letter *Dies Domini*, similarly draws from Jewish understandings of the Sabbath to inform the Christian observance of Sunday. Sunday, he argues, should be understood in the context of the biblical Sabbath, which he calls "a determining element in the kind of 'sacred architecture' of time which marks biblical revelation. It recalls that *the universe and history belong to God*; and without a constant awareness of that truth, man cannot serve in the world as co-worker of the Creator." (John Paul II 1998, section 1:15). For John Paul II, a Sabbath-inspired understanding of Sunday, which could include practices such as resting from work, reminds Christians that all time belongs to God and not to the marketplace. Many Christian theologians and spiritual writers have also framed Sabbath-keeping as a means to promote a "slower, simpler style of living," (see Hartman 2011, p. 58) to inspire the patronage of local food producers, and to encourage more intentional care for the natural environment (Hartman 2011, p. 59).

While these writers correctly see liturgical time, specifically Sabbath-keeping, as an important alternative to the modern temporal order, they often give little attention to strategies for collective praxis.[19] Many eschew the communal practice of resting from work on a fixed day of the week and advocate instead for do-it-yourself practices of individual rest and reflection.[20] Without a vision of collective action, such individualized practices could easily dissolve into the fragmentary, asynchronous framework of 24/7 temporality. These authors also appear not to recognize capitalism as the substratum that upholds the temporality they seek to transcend and resist, using instead terms such as "consumerism" that carry less critical weight.[21] When these authors neglect to diagnose capitalist ideology as the source of the present temporal regime, readers who follow them risk falling prey to the strategies of individualization and monetization key to the 24/7 project.

Two recent theologians have framed Sabbath-keeping as a mode of *collective* response to the 24/7 demands of late capitalism more explicitly than the authors previously mentioned. In his 2014 book, *Sabbath as Resistance: Saying No to the Culture of Now*, Walter Brueggemann frames a Sabbath spirituality of time as "an alternative to the endless demands of economic reality, more specifically the demands of market ideology." (Brueggemann 2017, p. xii). For Brueggemann, the present socio-economic order is akin to Pharaoh's regime in the book of Exodus. Keeping the Sabbath in imitation of the Israelites is how the people of God as a whole are witness to values higher than the insatiable urges of the market. The Sabbath, broadly understood, thus becomes an "occasion for reimagining all social life away from coercion and competition for compassionate solidarity." (Brueggemann 2017, p. 45). Brueggemann stresses that such solidarity is not achieved by sharing the mere idea of Sabbath-keeping; it requires concrete, shared liturgical, ethical, and economic praxis (Brueggemann 2017, p. 18).

Theologian Daniel Castillo has recently expanded upon Brueggemann's theologizing about the Sabbath to stress even more forcefully the importance of shared temporality for building habits of solidarity between various socio-economic groups and between human beings and the earth. Drawing from the tradition of liberation theology, Castillo argues that the regular, repeated practice of Sabbath-keeping (which can be read as gathering for worship on Sundays) should continuously challenge the community "to maintain its prophetic edge in negotiating with the globalization project's ways of organizing creation." (Castillo 2019, p. 208). Sabbath-keeping allows communities to "discern the times" in order to clarify the shape of religious and ethical–political praxis, to gather in community as a witness against the "fragmenting and isolating mechanisms" of late capitalism, and to celebrate in joyful hope of God's victory over the power of sin and death (Castillo 2019, pp. 210–11). Sabbath practices are necessary to achieve the goals of solidarity and liberative discipleship because such a difficult commitment must be constantly renewed, week by week (Castillo 2019, p. 207).

Brueggemann's and Castillo's understandings of the Sabbath improve upon previous articulations by naming capitalism explicitly and by framing liturgical praxis as a providing a temporal horizon for the cultivation of solidarity to defy the fragmentation and destruction of 24/7 temporality. However, like the other theologians of Sabbath mentioned above, they do not offer models for shared, collective praxis or explain why solidarity might take shape within this temporal framework. A spirituality of liturgical time that remains untethered to concrete, collective practices cannot sufficiently address the all-encompassing nature of 24/7 temporality. An articulation of a more robust praxis of liturgical time is needed, one that preserves and extends a liberative spirituality of the Sabbath.

4. Beyond the Sabbath: Liturgical Temporality as Time for Solidarity

For the remainder of this essay, I will propose that the Christian tradition possesses a rich liturgical spirituality and praxis of time that could provide a temporality in which to "learn to be contemporaneous together," to invoke Chan once again. With the embrace of a robust vision and praxis of liturgical temporality, communities could link the story of redemption as it unfolds in liturgical time with concrete, communal actions that build solidarity with marginalized persons and groups, and the natural world.[22] Ritual–liturgical practices, of course, cannot guarantee the outcomes one might desire from them. As Lauren Winner has recently argued, liturgical practices can not only form but also *de-form* in ways that are specific to the nature of those practices.[23] One possible de-formative function of keeping steadfastly to a robust liturgical temporality, precisely because it can provide a rich context for group formation, is to encourage exclusivism and triumphalism within the community.[24] For example, one can observe a tendency within some contemporary Orthodox Christian groups that strictly follow the Julian Calendar or "Old Calendar" to condemn and alienate other Orthodox and otherwise Christian groups that use the newer, Gregorian calendar, accusing them of error and even doctrinal heresy.[25] Nevertheless, liturgical temporality possesses unique features that can allow for solidarity to take shape within a wide-ranging and multi-layered temporal framework that counteracts certain deformative effects of 24/7 time.

Philosopher Christina Gschwandtner's recent book *Welcoming Finitude: Toward a Phenomenology of Orthodox Liturgy* gives an account of how liturgical temporality can work in the Orthodox Christian tradition, a tradition with an especially robust and vigorous tradition of liturgical time keeping throughout days, weeks, seasons, and years.[26] She draws from philosophers in the European tradition of phenomenology, especially Martin Heidegger, to explain how liturgical time can become the primary temporal horizon for a community's experience.[27] Gschwandtner's account demonstrates how liturgical temporality could provide a shared context for the cultivation of habits of solidarity in service of spiritual resistance to the destructive effects of 24/7 temporality. Below, I discuss three specific ways in which liturgical temporality could allow this to take shape.

First, liturgical temporality rejects an extractive attitude toward time. In 24/7 temporality, the individual inhabits a present that is largely indifferent to the past and moves into the future via the satiation of desires generated by ever-reloading stimuli and ever-new consumer products. Aided by the practice of systematic forgetting, extraction proceeds without witness to the destruction it causes. By contrast, the liturgical "now" is structured by remembrance of the past and hope for the future. Gschwandtner contends, "The liturgical present is only given meaningfully it if is precisely given at the same time and within the same moment as memory and anticipation." (Gschwandtner 2019, p. 45). Each day on the Orthodox liturgical calendar is peppered with commemorations of saints and historical events. Through commemoration, the past is meaningfully taken up into the temporal horizon of anamnetic remembrance and eschatological hope. The presence of the past in the liturgical present is felt especially strongly on major feasts such as the Nativity of Christ on December 25. One of the main Orthodox Christian hymns for the feast reads, "Today the Virgin gives birth to the Transcendent One,/and the earth offers a cave to the Unapproachable One!/Angels with shepherds glorify Him!/The wise men journey with a star!/Since for our sake the Eternal God was born as a Little Child!"[28] This hymn illustrates how, in liturgical temporality, the kairotic "today" straddles time and eternity, past and future. Gschwandtner writes, "Each moment matters profoundly, not as one in sequences of nows, but as the moment that encapsulates all of time. The heightened moment of the feast, then, in some way infects all of time, bleeds into the ordinary, and gives it significance."[29] Liturgy's temporal horizon of remembrance and hope is not limited to salvific events in the distant past but provides a context for remembering more recent events as well. This is critically important in the 24/7 age of systematic forgetting. Upon exiting the exhibition dedicated to the memory of the Holocaust at Yad Vashem, the Holocaust memorial center in New York, one reads, "Forgetfulness leads to exile, while remembrance is the secret of redemption." (Quoted in (Spiegel 2002, p. 156)). Forgetting has dire consequences, and a regular practice of remembrance must be cultivated to resist it. Liturgical temporality provides the context for such a practice.

Second, while 24/7 temporality militates against shared narratives in favor of fragmented, individual stories, liturgical temporality invites worshippers into a shared yet variegated story not of their own making. In liturgical time, "We are no longer the ones who open the world, but become dispossessed, swallowed up in the larger story."[30] Liturgical time is meaningful precisely because "we" did not invent it; it did not begin with us (Gschwandtner 2019, pp. 54–55). This temporal structure could allow for communities to cultivate solidarity by seeing themselves, others, and the earth as players in an ongoing story of salvation and liberation in Christ, looking forward to renewed heavens and a renewed earth. As Pope Francis writes, "Solidarity, understood in its most profound meaning, is a way of making history." (Francis 2020, para. 116). The Orthodox Christian liturgical year contains overlapping stories, cycling through moments in the lives of Christ, the Virgin Mary, and others. These dense narrative layers allow individuals to seek out healthy differentiation within the broader, shared story and identify with persons or events that relate to circumstances within one's own personal life and life together. The time of year that is shared most fully by all is Holy Week, the week preceding Pascha (Easter). Every year, this week is packed with worship services commemorating the final days before Jesus's death and resurrection. Such a schedule, Gschwandtner notes, "wreaks havoc on one's 'normal' schedule—one enters into a different kind of temporality where regular time seems suspended." (Gschwandtner 2019, p. 46). Many parishioners take time off from work to attend lengthy services. This time spent deep within the shared story of redemption is felt to matter more than other times because of the worshippers' anticipation of the Paschal feast. This feast involves both spiritual and material preparation—prayer, fasting, cooking, and cleaning—and is colored by memories of past feasting.[31] These communal practices can allow a spirit of solidarity and mutual aid to take shape as relationships grow and deepen. As people are guided by its rhythms of feasting and fasting, work and rest, liturgical temporality can gradually become the fabric of everyday life and lay claim to all time—season after season, year after year (Gschwandtner 2019, p. 49).

Finally, liturgical temporality thrives on meaningful repetition, which provides a context for the cultivation of habits of solidarity. As discussed above in Section 2 of this essay, the constant repetition of "new" yet functionally interchangeable digitally mediated experiences in 24/7 temporality was designed primarily for the extraction of maximum monetary value from time. The repetition at the heart of disaster capitalism, in the words of philosopher Maurice Blanchot, is "neither mournful nor nostalgic, the undesired return." (Blanchot 1986, p. 42). Rather than an endless repetition of novelty, the liturgy's repeated cycles of feasts, fasts, and commemorations allow communities to craft and appropriate a shared narrative arc of salvation, liberation, and human and non-human flourishing. Such an appropriation of a shared temporal horizon is not easy, nor is it guaranteed. Orthodox Christians sometimes complain of the repetitiveness and length of the services. Nonetheless, as Gschwandtner reminds the reader, one is shaped only by that which she puts her mind and body into. While ritual repetition can serve to perpetuate and enforce oppressive power structures, it can also allow for the formation of habits of solidarity when combined with educational, ethical, and other kinds of formation.[32] These habits could have a concrete, transformative effect on a community and its surroundings. One could determine the success or failure of a community's efforts to embrace liturgical temporality as a time for solidarity by examining certain changes over long periods of time. Such changes could include an increase in the level of the community's engagement in local neighborhoods and habitats, the integration of religious education—oriented around cycles of liturgical time—and community action toward solidarity, and changes in perceptions of the community by those around it. In other words, embracing such a vision and praxis of liturgical temporality could allow inward practices of devotion structured by liturgical time to extend outward, to concrete actions that foster solidarity and liberation from the destructive effects of late capitalist 24/7 temporality.

5. Conclusions

I have proposed that Christian traditions of liturgical temporality could provide a context for religious communities to cultivate solidarity between people of various classes, groups, and identities, and between human beings and the earth in resistance to the disaster capitalist regime of 24/7 temporality accelerated during the COVID-19 pandemic. Such solidarity within liturgical temporality is not a narrowly political form of resistance. To quote Blanchot, it is "spiritual resistance," a form of resistance without which political resistance is incomplete. He writes, "Resistance has no meaning, if not simply for oneself, or for the sake of friendship, which is rare. Only the religious have firm conviction capable of giving significance to life, and to death. Thus resistance is spiritual. Not until the revolts issuing from the depths ... do perspectives open—do ruined words become audible rising from the ruins, traversing the silence."[33] Incorporating yet expanding upon practices of the Sabbath, shared liturgical temporality should embrace the creative tension between rest and action, preparation and celebration, remembrance and hope, at the varied timescales of weeks, seasons, years, and lifetimes. Such a multifaceted and yet unified temporality, to quote Castillo, "undercuts the ideological homogenization of time and, instead, foregrounds the community's hope in the power of God to redeem history." (Castillo 2019, p. 207). While ultimate redemption and liberation remain just beyond the eschatological border of liturgical time, they are nevertheless already present, breaking in with each act of love, justice, and forgiveness.

Funding: This research received no external funding.

Conflicts of Interest: The author declares no conflict of interest.

Notes

1 See, e.g., (Bryson 2007; Derickson 2014; Veal 2019).
2 My understanding of the multivalency of solidarity in this paper is informed by Sobrino and Pico (1985). The authors write that solidarity is "another name for the kind of love that moves feet, hands, hearts, material goods, assistance, and sacrifice toward the pain, danger, misfortune, disaster, repression or death of other persons or a whole people ... The aim is to share with them and help them rise up, become free, claim justice, rebuild." (ibid., p. vii).
3 "Blursday" is not a neologism new to 2020; previously, it referred to a day spent hung over after a night of heavy drinking. See Alyeskyeyeva et al. (2020, p. 207). Craig D. Parks highlights the important role of social isolation due to virus prevention protocols in creating this disorienting sense of time. See Parks (2020, esp. p. 116).
4 Mathew Arthur aptly describes the digitally-mediated Blursday of the pandemic: "Time feels weird. The last two weeks have been a strange ten years. #blursday is pandemic coming into form as a feeling of time trending on Twitter. It stretches out the present with scope-creeping domesticities, hangovers, professionalisms, streaming video, and oversleep. Days collapse into a dark-mode user interface, online shopping cart grid, anxious infographic, or COVID-19 meme." (Arthur 2019–2020, p. x).
5 See, e.g., (Kohan 2021; 2020).
6 See Fottrell (2021). I do not wish to suggest that the effects of this trend are solely negative. One can see working from home as an opportunity, for example, to spend more time with family and friends, eating meals, etc., and less time commuting.
7 (Klein 2007). See also Lowrey (2020).
8 See Sagan (2019). Crary writes, "24/7 is inseparable from environmental catastrophe in its declaration of permanent expenditure, of endless wastefulness for its sustenance, in its terminal disruption of the cycles and seasons on which ecological integrity depends." (Crary 2013, p. 10).
9 (Crary 2013, p. 9). See also the classic article by Thompson (1967).
10 (Le Goff 1960); translation in ibid., Time, Work, and Culture in the Middle Ages (Chicago: University of Chicago Press, 1980), pp. 29–42
11 Crary writes, "The homogenizing force of capitalism is incompatible with any inherent structure of differentiation: sacred-profane, carnival-workday, nature-culture, machine-organism, and so on." (Crary 2013, p. 13).
12 (Crary 2013, p. 29). Crary further remarks that the late-capitalist goal is to transform "all users into interchangeable objects of the same mass dispossession of time and praxis." (ibid., p. 58). Sagan issues a useful critique of Crary's singular focus on the present by stressing the peculiar futurity of late-capitalist temporality, writing, "But another facet of the very same temporalities consists of speeds and constant subjection of the everyday to a never sated, futurist state of desire for more (more information, more technological and newer, soon-to-become-obsolete devices, etc.)." (Sagan 2019, p. 158).
13 (Chan 2020, p. 6). Emphasis added.
14 (Crary 2013, p. 57). Emphasis added.
15 Philosopher Maurice Blanchot, writing about disaster time, notes that the fragmentation of time amidst disaster does not allow for fixity, but rather "disarray [and] confusion." (Blanchot 1986, p. 7).
16 See, e.g., Odell (2019). The website The Nap Ministry advertises sleep as liberation and a means of clogging the gears of capitalist production and consumption. See https://thenapministry.wordpress.com/ (accessed on 7 May 2021). Both of these sources find inspiration in performance art for imagining alternative temporalities to 24/7 temporality.
17 For Heschel's partnership with Martin Luther King Jr. in organizing and activism, see Heschel (2018).
18 (Dawn 1989). For a critique of the notion of Sunday as Christian Sabbath, see Searle (1995).

19 Norman Wirzba recognizes, "It is important to realize that we will not be able to do this easily as individuals. Sabbath practices are corporate in nature, which means that we will need to enlist the help of others to keep us accountable and true to out better intentions." (Wirzba 2006, p. 151). However, he offers no communal strategies for the cultivation of Sabbath practice in a Christian context.

20 While many do discuss Sunday as a Christian Sabbath, they often criticize Puritan-inspired practices like work prohibition on Sundays, instead advocating practices of rest a regular day of the week that would, hopefully, influence the way in which one uses time throughout the rest of the week. See, e.g., Wirzba (2006, p. 91).

21 Consumerism is not co-terminus with capitalism, though they are obviously linked. It is important to note the extent to which the pursuit of desires, usually in the form of consumer goods, is intimately linked with corporate interests of maximum profitability in late capitalism. Theologian Kathryn Tanner puts it this way: "Whether at home, at the store, or at work, one should be the sort of person who assumes responsibility for making the most of what one has in pursuit of one's goals: the ever greater achievement of self-realization and self-fulfillment. Put into more financialized terms ... one should make every effort, in a self-directed way, to maximize the profitable employment of assets one has in one's person." (Tanner 2019, p. 73).

22 Such actions could include participating in local projects for fair housing and equitable access to healthy food and water, advocacy on behalf of residential areas disproportionately affected by pollution, protests, phone banking, and sit-ins for racial and environmental justice, and so on.

23 (Winner 2018). Winner critiques a prevalent, if mostly unspoken, assumption in postliberal theologies of practice that Christian practices always do what they are supposedly intended to do: form moral communities oriented towards virtue and sanctity. See (ibid., pp. 167–80).

24 Ritual theorist Catherine Bell notes, "Calendrical distinctions are effective in solidifying group identity, while the appropriation of local rites acts to extend that identity to new subgroupings." (Bell 1997, p. 105).

25 Such exclusivism around liturgical time can be understood, at least in part, as an effort to hold onto a sense of group identity in the midst of a changing world. See Demacopoulos (2017, esp. pp. 484–89).

26 (Gschwandtner 2019). Within the scholarly literature on ritual, time is a surprisingly neglected theme. One important exception is Roy Rappaport (1992). I have chosen to engage Gschwandtner as a primary conversation partner in this section because she is especially attentive to Christian ritual time in light of the Christianity's particular spiritual and ethical claims.

27 Gschwandtner describes liturgical temporality thus: "Instead of a linear experience that moves from past through the present to the future, time is experienced as the horizon within which we experience our liturgical being; it is the 'how' of our 'being' in its world." (Gschwandtner 2019, p. 44).

28 The Kontakion hymn for the Feast of Nativity on December 25 by the sixth-century hymn writer Romanos the Melodist. Translation from Orthodox Church in America, https://www.oca.org/saints/troparia/1000/12/25/103638-the-nativity-of-our-lord-god-and-savior-jesus-christ (accessed on 8 March 2021). For a perceptive discussion of time and communal identity in the hymns of Romanos, see Krueger (2014, pp. 66–105).

29 (Gschwandtner 2019, p. 55). It is important to mention that the Christian liturgical year developed in ancient and medieval temporal milieux foreign to modern notions of time as linear and quantifiable. One moves back and forth between past, present and future such that the modern worshipper might feel they are "time-travelling." But the point is that the present is subject to past and future, and is indeed structured by them. See the discussion in (ibid., pp. 43–45).

30 (Gschwandtner 2019, p. 46). She continues, "Our present reality is at the very least affected, possibly challenged and transformed by the liturgical reality that becomes present in our celebration of it." (ibid., p. 46).

31 (Gschwandtner 2019, p. 47). She continues, "We 'give up' other time—sometimes even quite inordinate amounts of time—in order to 'have the time' for celebration." (ibid., p. 48).

32 (Gschwandtner 2019, pp. 51–52). Ritual theorist Ronald Grimes wisely notes, "Rites may become not only irrelevant but oppressive. In the wrong hands, they can be tools for oppression as surely as they can be instruments of healing." See Grimes (2002, p. 293).

33 (Blanchot 1986, p. 83). See also Castillo (2019, p. 208).

References

Alyeskyeyeva, Iryna O., Tetyana A. Chaius, and Elizaveta A. Galitska. 2020. Coronaspeak as Key to Coronaculture: Studying New Cultural Practices Through Neologisms. *International Journal of English Linguistics* 10: 202–12.

Anonymous. 2020. Big Tech Companies, Fully Recovered from Pandemic, Report Record Earnings. *CBS News*. October 29. Available online: https://www.cbsnews.com/news/google-apple-amazon-facebook-twitter-big-tech-record-earnings-q3-2020/ (accessed on 7 March 2021).

Arthur, Mathew. 2019–2020. Writing Pandemic Feels. *Capacious: Journal for Emerging Affect Inquiry* 2: vi–xxiii.

Bell, Catherine. 1997. *Ritual: Perspectives and Dimensions*. Oxford: Oxford University Press.

Bell, Genevieve. 2021. Pandemic Passages: An Anthropological Account of Life and Liminality during COVID-19. *Anthropology in Action* 28: 79–84. [CrossRef]

Blanchot, Maurice. 1986. *The Writing of the Disaster*. Translated by Ann Smock. Lincoln, London: University of Nebraska Press.

Brueggemann, Walter. 2017. *Sabbath as Resistance: Saying No to the Culture of Now*, rev. ed. Louisville: Westminster John Knox Press.

Bryson, Valerie. 2007. *Gender and the Politics of Time: Feminist Theory and Contemporary Debates*. Bristol: Policy.

Castillo, Daniel P. 2019. *An Ecological Theology of Liberation: Salvation and Political Ecology*. Maryknoll: Orbis.

Chan, Nadine. 2020. Pandemic Temporalities: Distal Futurity in the Digital Capitalocene. *Journal of Environmental Media* 1: 1–8. [CrossRef]

Crary, Jonathan. 2013. *24/7: Late Capitalism and the Ends of Sleep*. London: Verso.

Dawn, Marva J. 1989. *Keeping the Sabbath Wholly: Ceasing, Resting, Embracing, Feasting*. Grand Rapids: Eerdmans.

Demacopoulos, George. 2017. 'Traditional Orthodoxy' as a Postcolonial Movement. *Journal of Religion* 97: 475–99. [CrossRef]

Derickson, Alan. 2014. *Dangerously Sleepy: Overworked Americans and the Cult of Manly Wakefulness*. Philadelphia: University of Pennsylvania Press.

Fottrell, Quentin. 2021. Will COVID-19 Push More Employees to Work Remotely after the Pandemic? This Economist Says Yes. *Marketwatch*. December 27. Available online: https://www.marketwatch.com/story/does-covid-19-have-the-power-to-revolutionize-work-this-economist-says-yes-2020-12-11 (accessed on 7 March 2021).

Francis. 2013. The Joy of the Gospel: Apostolic Exhortation, Evangelii Gaudium, of the Holy Father Francis to the Bishops, Clergy, Consecrated Persons and the Lay Faithful on the Proclamation of the Gospel in Today's World. Available online: http://www.vatican.va/content/francesco/en/apost_exhortations/documents/papa-francesco_esortazione-ap_20131124_evangelii-gaudium.html (accessed on 7 March 2021).

Francis. 2020. All Brothers: Encyclical Letter, Fratelli Tutti, of the Holy Father Francis on Fraternity and Social Friendship. Available online: http://www.vatican.va/content/francesco/en/encyclicals/documents/papa-francesco_20201003_enciclica-fratelli-tutti.html (accessed on 20 April 2021).

Grimes, Ronald L. 2002. *Deeply into the Bone: Re-Inventing Rites of Passage*. Berkeley: University of California Press.

Gschwandtner, Christina M. 2019. *Welcoming Finitude: Toward a Phenomenology of Orthodox Liturgy*. New York: Fordham University Press.

Hartman, Laura M. 2011. Christian Sabbath-keeping as a Spiritual and Environmental Practice. *Worldviews* 15: 47–64. [CrossRef]

Heschel, Abraham Joshua. 1951. *The Sabbath: Its Meaning for Modern Man*. New York: Farrar, Straus, and Young.

Heschel, Susannah. 2018. A Friendship in the Prophetic Tradition: Abraham Joshua Heschel and Martin Luther King Jr. *Telos* 182: 67–84. [CrossRef]

John Paul II. 1998. The Lord's Day: Apostolic Letter, Dies Domini, of the Holy Father John Paul II to the Bishops, Clergy and Faithful of the Catholic Church on Keeping the Lord's Day Holy. Available online: http://www.vatican.va/content/john-paul-ii/en/apost_letters/1998/documents/hf_jp-ii_apl_05071998_dies-domini.html (accessed on 7 March 2021).

Klein, Naomi. 2007. *The Shock Doctrine: The Rise of Disaster Capitalism*. New York: Picador.

Kohan, Shelley E. 2021. Amazon's Net Profit Soars 84% With Sales Hitting $386 Billion. *Forbes*. February 2. Available online: https://www.forbes.com/sites/shelleykohan/2021/02/02/amazons-net-profit-soars-84-with-sales-hitting-386-billion/ (accessed on 7 March 2021).

Krueger, Derek. 2014. *Liturgical Subjects: Christian Ritual, Biblical Narrative, and the Formation of the Self in Byzantium*. Philadelphia: University of Pennsylvania Press.

Le Goff, Jacques. 1960. Au Moyen Age: Temps de l'Eglise et temps du marchand. *Annales: Histoire, Sciences Sociales* 15: 417–33. [CrossRef]

Lowrey, Annie. 2020. Don't Blame Econ 101 for the Plight of Essential Workers. *The Atlantic*. May 13. Available online: https://www.theatlantic.com/ideas/archive/2020/05/why-are-americas-most-essential-workers-so-poorlytreated/611575/ (accessed on 7 March 2021).

Odell, Jenny. 2019. *How to do Nothing: Resisting the Attention Economy*. New York: Melville House.

Parks, Craig D. 2020. Group Dynamics When Battling a Pandemic. *Group Dynamics: Theory, Research, and Practice* 24: 115–21. [CrossRef]

Rappaport, Roy. 1992. Ritual, Time, and Eternity. *Zygon* 27: 5–30. [CrossRef]

Sagan, Claire. 2019. Capitalist Temporalities as Uchronia. *Theory & Event* 22: 143–74.

Searle, Mark. 1995. Sunday: The Heart of the Liturgical Year. In *Between Memory and Hope: Readings on the Liturgical Year*. Edited by Maxwell E. Johnson. Collegeville: Liturgical Press, pp. 59–76.

Sobrino, Jon, and Juan Hernández Pico. 1985. *Theology of Christian Solidarity*. Maryknoll: Orbis.

Spiegel, Gabrielle M. 2002. Memory and History: Liturgical Time and Historical Time. *History and Theory* 41: 149–62. [CrossRef]

Tanner, Kathryn. 2019. *Christianity and the New Spirit of Capitalism*. New Haven: Yale University Press.

Thompson, Edward P. 1967. Time, Work-Discipline, and Industrial Capitalism. *Past & Present* 38: 56–97.

Veal, Anthony James. 2019. *Whatever Happened to the Leisure Society?* Abingdon: Routledge.

Winner, Lauren F. 2018. *The Dangers of Christian Practice: On Wayward Gifts, Characteristic Damage, and Sin*. New Haven: Yale University Press.

Wirzba, Norman. 2006. *Living the Sabbath: Discovering the Rhythms of Rest and Delight*. Grand Rapids: Brazos Press.

religions

MDPI

Article

A "Liturgical Mysticism of Open Eyes": Johann Baptist Metz, Caryll Houselander, and Pandemic Liturgy

Samantha Slaubaugh

Department of Theology, University of Notre Dame, Notre Dame, IN 46556, USA; sslaubau@nd.edu

Abstract: The German theologian Johann Baptist Metz (1928–2019) called for a spirituality that sees more suffering, not less, the more liberated it is; he has described this as a "mysticism of open eyes." This theological vision involves all people, living and dead, becoming free to stand as subjects before God. Caryll Houselander (1901–1954), an English author, developed a liturgically infused mysticism focused on seeing Christ in each person. Her vision of Christ in others was rooted in creatively portraying the particularities of human life in the great "rhythm" of the Christ-life lived in the Mystical Body and expressed in the liturgy. This article proposes that juxtaposing these two authors reveals a "liturgical mysticism of open eyes," playing off Metz's initial phrasing. The work of Metz and Houselander together presents a fruitful liturgical theology for Christian communities during and in response to the pandemic as they engage questions of suffering, justice, and responsibility. By rooting our decisions about liturgical and social lives in a "liturgical mysticism of open eyes," the church may remain rooted to a liturgical spirituality, while also recognizing and being open to the suffering of individuals and communities while liturgies are altered, moved online, or postponed altogether.

Keywords: Johann Baptist Metz; Caryll Houselander; COVID-19; pandemic; social justice; suffering; oppression; liturgy; worship; ethics

1. Introduction

At first glance, there seems to be little in common between Johann Baptist Metz (1928–2019), the German priest and professional theologian known for political theology, and Caryll Houselander (1901–1954), the English lay theologian and artist known for liturgically infused work. However, each theologian was deeply marked by World War II, making a theology of the passion, or of compassion, a primary aspect of their work. Their experiences of mass death and suffering make both Metz and Houselander helpful sources of theology as the world reels from the loss of life and suffering caused by both the coronavirus pandemic and the oppression that flows from white supremacy and Western colonialism.[1] Reading the two together, moreover, further enriches the gaps in each author's thought. While Metz worked on political theology, he did not develop a liturgical and sacramental focus. Scholars such as (Morrill 2000) and (Eggemeier 2012) have taken up this lacuna in Metz, proposing other authors to complement Metz. Houselander, on the other hand, focused greatly on liturgy and sacramental life while saying much less on political theology. However, each author presents, through different approaches, a mystical theology of openness to the other in which the memory of Christ is brought to bear as an interpretive framework for both the present and the future. Metz's "mysticism of open eyes" combines with Houselander's liturgical mysticism into a "liturgical mysticism of open eyes," that challenges us today to make choices for our communities of faith through a rootedness in liturgy that does not distort the memory of Christ's passion. To support this claim, this essay first examines Metz's theological vision of a mysticism of open eyes. Second, it looks at key themes in Houselander's liturgically rooted mystical theology. Finally, the essay concludes with questions aimed to interrupt our practice of liturgy in light of both the coronavirus pandemic and concerns for social justice. These interrupting questions invite us to consider how a solidaristic liturgy looks in our particular communities as we wrestle with racism, death, and physical and emotional suffering in a pandemic.

2. Johann Baptist Metz: "Mysticism of Open Eyes"

To begin a fruitful juxtaposition of Metz and Houselander, one should start first with an exploration of what Metz envisioned in the phrase "mysticism of open eyes." Metz argued that "Jesus did not teach an ascending mysticism of closed eyes, but rather a God-mysticism with an increased readiness for perceiving, a mysticism of open eyes, which sees more and not less. It is a mysticism that especially makes visible all invisible and inconvenient suffering, and—convenient or not—pays attention to it and takes responsibility for it, for the sake of a God who is a friend to human beings" (Metz 1998, p. 163). For Metz, a true mysticism, one in which a person enters the mystery of their own existence as a subject in God's presence, is always a mysticism that sees more of life and not less. Metz was not interested in a mystical "opium" in which those uncomfortable with the pain and suffering of the world escape to an ethereal experience of oblivion before God. Rather, to be a subject before God is to be a "witness," one who is "involved, with eyes that see, in that history where people are crucified and tortured, hated and miserly loved;" for as Metz argues, only in "how we deal with others ... can it be known how we think about God and what we think of God" (Metz 1998, p. 163). Simply put, a "mysticism of open eyes" is "a mysticism of an unconditional obligation to feel the suffering of others" (Metz 2005, p. 32).

Metz's approach to articulating a Christian mysticism reaches to the core of his own practical fundamental theology. For Metz, theology is "mystical-political" (Metz 2007, p. 29); that is, theology is never merely pure doctrine dressed up later in praxis and narrative. Theology is always both practical and fundamental. Praxis and doctrine are intertwined and misunderstood when separated from each other. Metz articulated this succinctly when he argued that "Christ must always be thought in such a way that he is not just thought.... every Christology is nourished by a praxis: the praxis of discipleship" (Metz 2007, p. 62). This discipleship must be understood as a praxis of suffering since it cannot be achieved apart from Christ's own command to "pick up your cross and follow me."

Praxis as suffering is not masochistic but liberating; "the history of suffering [is] a history of freedom" (Morrill 2000, p. 31). The willingness to see more suffering and to have a mysticism of open eyes is a type of resistance to apathy. This praxis extends from a Christology that flows first and foremost from the cross; therefore, a mysticism of open eyes is a mysticism that sees the doctrine of Christology flowing from the "dangerous" memory of Christ's passion, death, and resurrection. Metz explained that this memory "holds a particular anticipation of the future as a future for the hopeless, the shattered and oppressed. In this way it is a dangerous and liberating memory, which badgers the present and calls it into question" (Metz 2007, p. 89). As dangerous as this memory is—for it takes one away from the safe, distant God who has little practical impact—it is fundamentally a liberative memory. The ability to remember this dangerous narrative of God coming into the world, suffering, and rising again frees one to see with open eyes the very narrative itself in one's own particular social and historical context. Metz's own thought is characterized by the need to take his own witness of suffering "not to the psychologist but into the church" (Metz 1998, p. 2). During World War II, upon returning from delivering a message, Metz found his whole company dead; he began to ask, "what would happen if ... one did not allow oneself to be talked out of such unreconciled memories even by theology, but rather wanted to have faith with them and, with them, speak about God?" (Metz 1998, p. 2). As the death of others was a foundational event for Metz's theological thought, he understands a mysticism of suffering to be rooted not in "a self-referential memory of suffering (the root of all conflicts!), but in the form of a memory of others' suffering, in the form of a remembrance of the stranger's suffering" (Metz 2005, p. 33).

In addition to the memory of suffering, the memory of Christ's passion, death, and resurrection, Metz also focused on two other concepts that illuminate a mysticism of open eyes, namely, narrative and solidarity.[2] As for narrative, Metz claimed that "[t]he logos of the cross and of the resurrection has an indispensable narrative structure. Confronted with the human history of suffering, faith ... is passed on in dangerous-liberating stories, under the impact of which those hearers who are affected by them become 'doers of the word'" (Metz 2007, p. 194). By narrating one's own world into the narrative of the dangerous memory of Christ's passion, death, and resurrection, the creedal and doctrinal content of faith becomes "understood as formulas in which this challenging remembrance is spelled out publicly" (Metz 2007, p. 89). Proclaiming the dangerous memory of Christ in history requires liberated mystical sight, as this sight is the way to true solidarity with all people, and thus the way for every person to become free to be subjects. This is the "task given to religion," according to Metz, namely, "to stand up so that all persons might be subjects in solidarity, just as much when confronted by violent oppression as in the face of the caricature of solidarity found in formed massification and in institutionalized hatred" (Metz 2007, p. 59).[3] Metz holds in tension a critique of privatization that results from the Enlightenment and the opposite extreme of "massification," or the "abstract negation of the individual" (Metz 2007, p. 59). To be a subject before God is to stand before God fully as oneself, related always and already to all other subjects. The individual is always unique, but always also realized in communion. The paradox of particularity and universality is a constant thread woven throughout Metz's vision of a "mysticism of open eyes" which sees the universality of the dangerous memory of Christ always in its particular iterations in history.[4]

Every historical and social context must be viewed through and integrated into this narrative of the dangerous memory. As such, a mysticism of open eyes is a mysticism of interruption. The suffering of others, convenient or not, interrupts our understanding of the narrative and asks pointed questions about one's own and one's community's responsibility and response to the memory of the passion, death, and resurrection that is being lived out in a given time and place. This mysticism of open eyes is intertwined with the praxis of discipleship, what Metz called a "practical Christ-formedness" which is the sign of the Spirit at work (Metz 2007, p. 155). Although brief, this summary of Metz's mysticism of open eyes should be enough to offer a comparison with Houselander's own theology. However, two final points are important to highlight.

First, the solidarity implicated in a mysticism of open eyes extends even to the dead who have been vanquished and forgotten. Metz argued that solidarity is "expanded into an anamnestic solidarity, a solidarity of memory with the victims of history" (Metz 2007, p. 68). The dead victims of history are exemplary of the type of solidarity Metz proposed is required by a mysticism of open eyes; "when it comes to the dead there is no exchange relationship ... The love that mourns for the dead is that form of love ... that cannot be taken up into a consumer society's exploitation structures" (Metz 2007, p. 51). The dead have nothing to offer the living from a consumer standpoint. Yet, the eschatological content of the memory of Christ's passion, death, and resurrection makes space in particular for the dead, who are promised resurrection. Therefore, a mysticism of open eyes sees not only the living who suffer, but also the dead who have suffered and been forgotten. This solidarity interrupts and shapes an eschatological understanding of the hoped-for future.

Second, the praxis of solidarity is well-expressed in prayer, in which one is free to stand as a subject before God in solidarity with all people, not as a privatized individual. While Metz did not expound in depth on liturgy, ritual, and sacrament—what Matthew Eggemeier calls "distinctive lacunae" (Eggemeier 2012, p. 54)—his own theological project dovetails naturally with liturgical theology. Bruce Morrill has demonstrated this point by placing Metz and Alexander Schmemenn in conversation (Morrill 2000). Moreover, prayer, ritual, and sacrament are not in contradiction to Metz's theological vision, though they are subject to manipulation by bourgeois religion. Metz was concerned with liturgy that enables a spirituality of closed eyes. He argued that a liberated spirituality "cannot be limited to a purely cultic experience, isolated from and unburdened by conflicts, repression, and challenges in everyday life" (Metz 2007, p. 93). In contrast with a "purely cultic" spirituality, Metz envisioned a church that "has an ear for the dark prophecy of this suffering of others" (Metz 2007, p. 94). Moreover, Metz did call for the integration of "the sacramental event into stories of life and of suffering ... [to] make it clear that the sacramental event is a narrative of salvation within these stories" (Metz 2007, p. 190). Not only is liturgy relevant to Metz's work due to its narrative structure of proclaiming the dangerous memory of Christ, but in prayer God "calls us to become subjects or unconditionally support others becoming subjects ... and [God] calls us to remain subjects in the face of guilt and in opposition both to the dissolution of individual identity into 'the masses' and also to apathy" (Metz 2007, p. 80). Prayer is the place in which we narrate the memory of Christ in solidarity with all; that is true even especially if we bear guilt or responsibility for the oppression that takes away another's freedom to be subjects before God. Liturgy is where the history of the vanquished, not the conquerors, and the guilt and responsibility of the church must be proclaimed as interruptions to our liturgical theology and praxis, or else we will not be free to stand as subjects in solidarity before God.

3. Caryll Houselander: Liturgical Mysticism

Turning now to Caryll Houselander's articulation of mysticism, solidarity, and liturgy, both similarities and differences between her and Metz will become apparent. Houselander's mystical theology is captured by her description of three visionary experiences detailed in her autobiography, *A Rocking-Horse Catholic*. In the first vision at the beginning of World War I, she saw an ostracized Bavarian nun crying; Houselander looked down in embarrassment and when she looked back up, she saw the nun wearing the crown of thorns (Houselander 1988, p. 74). The nun whose nationality made her an enemy during the war was revealed as one participating in the passion of Christ. During the second vision in 1918, she saw an icon of Christ the King crucified floating in the sky; she later discovered that the vision of Christ had the face of the executed Russian Tsar, Nicholas II (Houselander 1988, p. 111). Houselander explained how this vision taught her that Christ's life was even lived by the wealthy and powerful. The third vision occurred when Houselander boarded a full underground train. She described how "quite suddenly I saw with my mind .... Christ in them all. ... not only was Christ in every one of them, living in them, dying in them, rejoicing in them, sorrowing in them—but because He was in them, and because they were here, the whole world was here too. ... not only all the people in all the countries of the world, but all those people who had lived in the past, and all those yet to come" (Houselander 1988, pp. 137–38). Houselander highlighted the theological broadening of these visions, stating that her third vision "was not a seeing of Christ in one person, as it had been with the Bavarian nun, or in one particular sort of person, as it had been in the living icon of Christ the King. This time it was Christ in all" (Houselander 1988, p. 137). Finding Christ in all people and situations was the core of Houselander's theological project.

After her mystical experience, she captured this mysticism of open eyes in her theological and creative work. While Metz's articulation of the mysticism of open eyes is best understood through the categories of memory, narrative, and solidarity, Houselander's used the themes of creativity, rhythm, and the Christ-life. First, moving beyond narrative, Houselander affirmed all creative work is integral to the structure of theology. In *The Risen Christ*, she described Christ as the archetypal artist who creates out of overflowing love in the Trinity; therefore, "we can all be artists and creators: in our attitude to our work we can make what we make first of all for love" (Houselander 1958, p. 84). Second, integral to the ideal of creativity is Houselander's concept of "rhythm." She did not describe her poetry as poems but as "rhythms." She wrote to a friend that "I have for a long time felt that a kind of communion of contemplation among us all is what is needed in the world, and I deliberately write Rhythms and give them to all sorts of people in order to start some recollection in their souls" (Houselander 1945, "From a Letter to Maisie Ward"). Rather than letting prayer take her out of the world, the Rhythms were a way in which Houselander brought the world into her prayer. Similar to Metz, she envisioned a spirituality that was not an ascending escape from suffering, but one in which God descends to the world, present even in its mundane experiences as a Rhythm that beats from the life, passion, death, and resurrection of Christ.

Third, Houselander argued that human life partakes in the one life of Christ, the artist whose rhythm of love unites all creation. In *This War is the Passion*, written about World War II, she claimed that "because [Christ] has made us 'other Christs,' because his life continues in each one of us, there is nothing that any one of us can suffer which is not the passion he suffered. Our redemption, although it was achieved completely by our Lord, does, by a special loving mercy of his, go on in us. It is one unbroken act which goes on in the mystical body of Christ on earth, which we are" (Houselander 2008, p. 1). The Christ-life is not so much an *imitatio Christi* that is accomplished by one's own effort, but rather, as in Houselander's third mystical vision, it is Christ himself living mystically in each individual. What is required, according to Houselander, is simply to learn to recognize the Christ-life being lived not only in one's own life, but in the life of each person. In other words, we must have open eyes to the suffering of Christ lived in the world. Similar to Metz, Houselander did not see Christ's universal presence in humanity as leading toward some unnamed mass of people that we are called to think about. Rather, both authors are clear that the universal and the particular are met in Christ, neither confused nor divided. Christ is in all but uniquely in each.

Parallel to the two notes on Metz's work, I wish to highlight two aspects of Houselander's thought. First, while Metz privileged the dead, Houselander privileged children and infants, another category of humanity that are often forgotten as real subjects. A survey of Houselander's work reveals that while she spent a great deal of time on the passion of Christ, the life of the Christ-child, both in actual children and in adults, is a primary theme. The two are not separate moments as much as they are the beginning and end of a circle; as Houselander put it, "Bethlehem is the inscape of Calvary" (Houselander [1949] 1995, p. 69). Houselander taught that all are to become as little children by living the Christ-child life, by which she envisioned, "we must get back true values instead of those that are based on materialism, public opinion, and snobbery; ... we must regain simplicity and humility ... we must become makers and poets again" (Houselander [1949] 1995, p. 87). Houselander emphasized that being subjects before God requires us to become as the Christ-child, which is deeply related not only to creativity but also to a praxis of suffering. "If the infant Christ is fostered in us, no life is trivial. No life is impotent before suffering, no suffering is too trifling to heal the world, too little to redeem, to be the point at which the world's healing begins" (Houselander [1949] 1995, p. 101). Houselander's focus on children is best understood as a way to see Christ in the suffering of those who have the least to contribute to society and are thus ignored or forgotten.

Second, unlike Metz, Houselander's mysticism is explicitly related to the liturgical and sacramental life of the church. Houselander taught that "the Liturgy is the expression of Christ's love, his prayer in his Mystical Body, into which our own prayer is gathered and integrated" (Houselander 1958, p. 68). Liturgy is also "the supreme expression on earth of the rhythmic Law of God" (Houselander [1949] 1995, p. 43). Unlike Metz, who mostly gestures provocatively toward the necessity of expounding upon the narrative structure in the liturgical and sacramental life of the church, Houselander actively narrated both the life of the world into the liturgy and the liturgy into the life of the world. "Houselander describes everyday occurrences in her life using the vocabulary of the liturgical rites of the church" (Petrin 2020, p. 224). In a rhythm titled "Low Mass on Sunday," Houselander affirmed a mysticism of open eyes that is rooted in the communion of the faithful:

> They are not more blessed
> whose feet
> are set on the mountain path,
> who abide in the cloud,
> content with the touch
> of a God who is featureless,
> than we
> who, weaker in faith,
> learn by touching His wounds
> in the human race
> that our hands
> touch with His power to heal:
> than we, at the wedding
> of earth and Heaven,
> turning the water to wine
> by a fling of the heart
> to God—
> in the lowliest,
> in the nearest at hand.
> We are the simple bread
> ground for the simpler Host.
> (Houselander 1945, p. 36)

Christ is not present in the host as if it were the hidden, featureless face of Christ in a cloud of darkness. Rather, the communion at mass is the communion of the people; they are the grain ground, baked, and broken together into the host, into Christ. "It is the breaking of the Bread which is the Communion of all [humans] in Christ, in which the multiple lives of the world are one Christ-life, the fragmentary sorrows of the world are one Christ-Passion" (Houselander [1949] 1995, p. 148). For Houselander, the liturgy was foundational for living a life with eyes open to see Christ in others. In this sense, I follow Eggemeier's lead in drawing upon other authors to illuminate what embodied practices form individuals, and in this case, entire communities, to not only see but also respond to the suffering of the world. Eggemeier discusses Sarah Coakley and Simone Weil as authors who argue for the role of contemplative prayer as a tool for responding to suffering; contemplation trains us to pay attention (Eggemeier 2012, pp. 54–57). In a similar vein, Houselander's work points to embodied practices missing in Metz's articulation of a "mysticism of open eyes." The liturgy opens our eyes, trains us to pay attention, and invites our bodies to participate in that dangerous memory of the passion, death, and resurrection of Christ. To read Metz and Houselander together, then, is to find a "liturgical mysticism of open eyes".

4. Conclusions: Questions for Liturgical Theology and Praxis in Light of the Pandemic

Turning then to our current situation, what might reading Metz and Houselander together contribute to our liturgical theology and praxis during a time when inequality in our society has been highlighted in so many ways? According to Metz, a mysticism of open eyes is a liberation that allows one to stand in true solidarity with others by means of the narrative of the dangerous memory of the passion, death, and resurrection of Jesus. According to Houselander, a liturgical mysticism is to see and then creatively proclaim the life, passion, death, and resurrection of Christ as told by the liturgy in the lives of every individual. Combining Metz's political theology with Houselander's liturgical theology leads to a "liturgical mysticism of open eyes." The liturgy is the place in which we publicly remember the dangerous memory of Christ's passion, death, and resurrection in order to have our eyes opened by God's grace to see the Christ-life in others. The implications of grounding our faith communities in a liturgical mysticism of open eyes are going to differ depending on the ecclesial and local community and thus cannot be fleshed out here with any completeness. Instead, I wish to ask a handful of questions that might helpfully interrupt our liturgical theology and begin to explore how answers to these questions might empower our liturgical praxis to publicly proclaim the dangerous memory of the Christ-life being lived in and around us.

First, are the most forgotten persons and those suffering the most in society the ones at the core of our theological understanding of Christ in the liturgy? If we follow Metz and Houselander, decisions about safety precautions in a pandemic must be made with a primary focus on the impact of these decisions for those whom society pushes to the margins and those who have been deprived of the power to prevent their own suffering from disease or injustice. It has become evident that those generally marginalized by systems of oppression are those who are suffering at a higher rate and with greater consequence from COVID-19.[5] The making and enforcement of safety decisions, such as masking, social distancing, or outdoor and online worship, must be made for the sake of those neglected by society, whether they be in the pews or not. Furthermore, these decisions must be communicated in such a way that it invites and empowers congregants to see the suffering caused by the pandemic as a narrative of Christ's passion and death. Our catechesis on these decisions should open eyes to see the mystical presence of Christ in those who suffer behind hospital curtains, nursing home doors, factory walls, and redlined neighborhoods. In practice, this might mean holding pastoral listening sessions with congregants who are upset about safety precautions put in place; it might result in tailoring sermons to such catechetical purposes; it might entail virtual communications that mystagogically interpret new liturgical symbols such as the space between congregants, the computer screen, masks, spiritual communion, and a lack of singing.[6]

Additionally, with an understanding that those who suffer injustice and oppression are at the heart of the liturgy and that they have a unique authority to witness to the memory of the passion, death, and resurrection of Christ, ministry teams and parishioners alike ought to actively listen to the voices of those risking their lives to, suffering, and dying from COVID-19, racism, and all forms of disasters and systemic oppression. Churches ought to be consistently centering these marginalized and suffering voices with the understanding that the proclamation of the gospel cannot stand apart from their witness and active contribution. Thus, churches should also examine their visible liturgies. Who do people see in the pews? Who do they see in leadership? Who do they see in the artwork that adorns the space, be it virtual or physical? Who are we missing at our eucharistic table, in our ordained and lay leadership, and in our proclamation of the gospel? Is the liturgical setting excluding those on the margins or is it re-centered around them? A liturgical mysticism of open eyes should flow from and lead to a visible performance of the liturgy that symbolizes its eschatological hope of liberation and redemption through art, lay and clerical performance, and text.

Second, are we turning to liturgies to creatively protest injustice and memorialize the dead? Houselander especially challenges our churches to embrace the creative aspect of liturgy flowing from God the Artist. Therefore, making changes due to safety precautions should be viewed as an opportunity to perform and creatively narrate the memory of the passion, death, and resurrection of Christ in a pandemic. If liturgy is a public proclamation of this dangerous memory, can more outdoor liturgies and public services that are not eucharistic (therefore avoiding exclusion around the Eucharist) aid in this proclamation? Gathering safely outdoors would be a public performance of the church's active response to the witness of suffering in the pandemic. Moreover, churches should be striving to draw from the liturgical riches of tradition in meeting the crisis of death and suffering caused by the pandemic and oppression of all kinds. Churches have long held a unique societal role in remembering and praying for the dead. Congregations can turn to their tradition's liturgical repertoire, adapting these liturgies when necessary, and perform liturgies in memory of all who have died during this pandemic. Whether this be requiem masses, the office of the dead, or memorial services, celebrating these liturgies as the church could act both as a liturgical reminder to parishioners to see the dead and the suffering and also as a public service for the mourning community. Additionally, with a vast history of processional liturgies and call-and-response litanies, Christian churches have the tools to mystagogically interpret protests for justice as a liturgical act. Moreover, the church can actively utilize outdoor processions to safely perform memorials for the dead and petitions for those suffering injustice, perhaps processing to local memorial sites, around hospitals, places of racial violence, or prominent public places. The physical movement of diverse bodies coming together and marching forward has potential to be both therapeutic in healing divisions and also prophetic in their public petitions to God for injustices to be made right.

Third, and finally, do we encourage worshipping communities to stand as subjects before God by not rejecting our guilt and the responsibility that follows true solidarity? Both public health measures and efforts for racial justice have encountered pushback inside the church. However, confession is an integral part of nearly every liturgy, not to mention a sacrament in several denominations. Christians then, should be equipped through their liturgical formation to clearly and humbly acknowledge their sins, both communal and personal. Our liturgies might better reflect this need to accept the guilt and responsibility that flows from solidarity with the suffering by adding or editing an invitation to confession that addresses the church's role in profiting from or causing oppression and suffering in the world, including through racism, colonialism, climate change, abuses of power, etc.[7] Our petitions can also reflect an outward concern for justice and an inward desire for our own communal turning from sin and to God. The sending out at the end of many liturgies too, might better reflect our current situation and be a specific call to fight for justice in our communities given our own eucharistic liberation from sin. The rhythm of the Christian liturgy from confession to communion to mission into the world invites the church to stand in solidarity, unafraid of their own guilt. God's mercy meets us, redeems us, and sends us into the world to perform communal penance as we fight for justice and take responsibility for injustices. Beyond eucharistic liturgies, could public liturgies of repentance for the church's own complicity in systems of oppression be formative for congregants and offer those harmed by the church a step toward full justice?

If we listen to Metz and Houselander, our liturgical theology and praxis will flow from our answers to these questions, and our answers must be formed by centering and listening to those who are suffering most in this pandemic. When this work begins, our liturgies will strive to reject a false peace without justice; they will turn from a privatized cultic experience where individuals are severed from a communion of solidarity. In the face of suffering and inequality, the liturgy should challenge us to open our eyes to the dangerous memory of the passion, death, and resurrection in the vanquished, forgotten, and oppressed; it should be where we creatively work in solidarity to shape our hope for the future in light of the Christ-life being revealed in the present.

Funding: This research received no external funding.

Conflicts of Interest: The author declares no conflict of interest.

Notes

1 For an English introduction to the work of Metz, see (Ashley 1998). The scholarship on Metz is significant; Houselander is much less studied. Ward (1962) is a well-known biography, and there are several academic

articles looking at Houselander's writings such as Coulter (1990), Meconi (2014), Meszaros (2015), and Petrin (2020).

2 These are not the only two themes relevant to a full understanding of Metz's work, of course. For an overview of Metz's six "central elements" in *Faith in History and Society*, see (Morrill 2000, pp. 21–26).

3 See (Vento 2002) for an analysis of how Metz's focus on suffering can contribute to feminist theology in light of violence against women and the resulting necessary political resistance.

4 For example, in the "biographical itinerary" that precedes *A Passion for God*, Metz explains: "I have worked to formulate a concept of theology that, while it recognizes the post-modernists' legitimate suspicion of universalistic approaches, does not collapse into a sheer relativization of cultural worlds. I have striven to do this by stressing a respect for and obedience to the authority of those who suffer. For me this authority is the only one in which the authority of the sovereign God is manifested in the world for all men and women" (Metz 1998, p. 4).

5 The Centers for Disease Control and Prevention, for example, indicate that "Race and ethnicity are risk markers for other underlying conditions that affect health, including socioeconomic status, access to health care, and exposure to the virus related to occupation" (CDC 2021).

6 Houselander herself engaged in this catechesis in *This War is the Passion*, giving a step-by-step method for spiritually praying the mass should it not be available during the bombings of London. Her catechesis focuses on lay participation, stating that the mass "is not a sacrifice offered by a priest in which our part is merely that of a devout audience. It is a sacrifice which gathers every circumstance of our life to itself and is the very core of our being" (Houselander 2008, p. 90).

7 See (Ramshaw 2017) for examples of laments on "Disease and Infirmity" (p. 22), "Injustices in Society" (p. 23), and "Damage to the Earth" (p. 24).

References

Ashley, James Matthew. 1998. *Interruptions: Mysticism, Politics, and Theology in the Work of Johann Baptist Metz*. Notre Dame: University of Notre Dame Press.

CDC—Center for Disease Control and Prevention. 2021. Risk for COVID-19 Infection, Hospitalization, and Death by Race/Ethnicity. Available online: https://www.cdc.gov/coronavirus/2019-ncov/covid-data/investigations-discovery/hospitalization-death-by-race-ethnicity.html (accessed on 14 July 2012).

Coulter, Moureen. 1990. 'A Mirror Set before the Face of God,' Art and Mysticism in the Work of Caryll Houselander. *Studia Mystica* 13: 83–95.

Eggemeier, Matthew T. 2012. A Mysticism of Open Eyes: Compassion For A Suffering World And The Askesis Of Contemplative Prayer. *Spiritus: A Journal of Christian Spirituality* 12: 43–62. [CrossRef]

Houselander, Caryll. 1945. *The Flowering Tree*. New York: Sheed and Ward.

Houselander, Caryll. 1958. *The Risen Christ*. New York: Sheed and Ward.

Houselander, Caryll. 1988. *A Rocking Horse Catholic*. Westminster: Christian Classics, Inc.

Houselander, Caryll. 1995. *Wood of the Cradle, Wood of the Cross. The Little Way of the Infant Jesus*. Manchester: Sophia Institute Press. First published 1949. *The Passion of the Infant Christ*. New York: Sheed and Ward.

Houselander, Caryll. 2008. *This War is the Passion*. Notre Dame: Christian Classics.

Meconi, David Vincent. 2014. Two Apostles of Loneliness: Caryll Houselander and Catherine Doherty on the Mystical Body of Christ. *Logos: A Journal of Catholic Thought and Culture* 17: 58–76. [CrossRef]

Meszaros, Julia. 2015. The Doctrine of 'Divine Indwelling' in Elizabeth of the Trinity and Caryll Houselander. *New Blackfriars* 96: 465–80. [CrossRef]

Metz, Johann Baptist. 1998. *A Passion for God: The Mystical-Political Dimension of Christianity*. Translated by J. Matthew Ashley. Mahwah: Paulist Press.

Metz, Johann Baptist. 2005. God: Against the Myth of the Eternity of Time. In *The End of Time? The Provocation of Talking about God*. Translated by J. Matthew Ashley. Mahwah: Paulist Press.

Metz, Johann Baptist. 2007. *Faith in History and Society: Toward a Practical Fundamental Theology*. Translated by J. Matthew Ashley. New York: The Crossroad Publishing Company.

Morrill, Bruce. 2000. *Anamnesis as Dangerous Memory: Political and Liturgical Theology in Dialogue*. Collegeville: The Liturgical Press.

Petrin, Anna Adams. 2020. Insights from Mrs. Murphy: Caryll Houselander as Liturgical Theologian. *Worship* 94: 206–27.

Ramshaw, Gail. 2017. *Pray, Praise, and Give Thanks: Litanies, Laments, and Thanksgivings at Font and Table*. Minneapolis: Augsburg Fortress.

Vento, Johann M. 2002. Violence, Trauma, and Resistance: A Feminist Appraisal of Metz's Mysticism of Suffering unto God. *Horizons* 29: 7–22. [CrossRef]

Ward, Maisie. 1962. *Caryll Houselander. That Divine Eccentric*. New York: Sheed and Ward.

religions

MDPI

Article

Spiritual Communion in a Digital Age: A Roman Catholic Dilemma and Tradition

Edward Foley

Catholic Theological Union, Chicago, IL 60615, USA; foley@ctu.edu

Abstract: In the midst of this pandemic, most Christian Churches in the United States have been required to limit severely if not suspend face-to-face worship. The responses to this challenge when it comes to celebrating the Eucharist have been multiple. Frequent pastoral responses have included the shipping of consecrated elements to folk for their use during live-stream worship and virtual communion, in which worshippers employ elements from their own households as communion elements during the digitized worship. These options are not permitted for Roman Catholics. Instead, it is most common for Roman Catholics to be invited into spiritual communion. This is often considered a diminished, even ternary form of communing, quickly dispensed when quarantines are lifted and herd immunity achieved. On the other hand, there is a rich and thoughtful tradition about spiritual communion that recognizes it as an essential element in communion even when such is experienced face-to-face. This article intends to affirm the values of spiritual communion as a real, mystical and fruitful action that not only sustains people worshipping from afar, but enhances an authentic eucharistic spirituality.

Keywords: virtual communion; live-streamed worship; pandemic; liturgy; spiritual communion

1. Introduction

The COVID-19 pandemic has wrought havoc on innumerable aspects of life. From this author's context in the United States, notable examples of such disruption are apparent in our educational systems, small business ventures, new stresses on the underemployed, and profound challenges to age cohorts, economic classes, or communities of color that have confronted multiple health and heath care issues for decades. Institutionalized religions, like my own Roman Catholicism, have also faced unforeseen challenges. Traditional forms of community building with their multiple strategies for gathering the faithful have either been banned outright or seriously restricted. Expected and deeply honored forms of pastoral care such as visiting and anointing the sick, hearing confessions, or accompanying the dying have similarly been reduced and in many situations eliminated. Other sacramental expectations—confirmed in our Code of Canon Law (1983), which acknowledges that the baptized have a right to the sacraments (can. 213)—have been delayed or denied. These include baptisms, marriage rites and funeral liturgies. The widest impact has been experienced around the still obligatory and spiritually important practice of Sunday Mass. While all relevant studies acknowledge the decline in weekly Mass attendance by Roman Catholics (e.g., Gambino 2019), the desire for Sunday worship and its culminating act of receiving the consecrated elements in communion is yet strong and documentable.

In response, many parishes have turned to livestreaming Sunday worship through Facebook, YouTube, or other digital venues. There are yet to be any wide-ranging empirical studies on exactly how many congregations are capable of providing this service. Anecdotal information clearly points to congregations more urban, white and financially stable as typically capable and inclined to providing such services. Furthermore, at this early stage, we do have sufficient data to understand how this virtual move has sustained, increased, or decreased engagement among the faithful, much less good data about the quality of that engagement. At one parish in which I preside and preach, the pre-COVID-19 practice of live streaming the 5:00 p.m. Mass on Sunday afternoon would draw around 300 hits (Old St. Patrick's Church n.d., 4667723). The first Sunday during the shuttering of churches, admittedly adjacent to its highly touted patronal feast day, the parish combined its St. Patrick's celebration with its first livestreamed 10:00 a.m. Mass, garnering 36,502 viewers (Old St. Patrick's Church n.d., 9038563).

While a preliminary analysis of such anecdotal information suggests that the digital availability of Sunday and even weekday Mass is of great value to many, it also triggers a particular dilemma. A theological as well as experiential highpoint of the Mass for many Roman Catholics is reception of communion, especially the bread. A hallmark of the 20th century liturgical reforms was the promotion of more frequent communion among the faithful. This began with the reforms of Pius X (d. 1914), who lowered the age requirement for communion from 12 to 7 years of age (*Quam Singulari*, Pius X 1910). It continued through the reforms of Pius XII (d. 1958), who twice modified the fasting requirements before communion (*Christus Dominus*, Pius XII 1953 and *Sacram Communionem*, Pius XII 1957). This eucharistic promotion culminated in Vatican II's 1963 decree on the liturgy, which considers the faithful's reception of the eucharist the "more perfect form of participation in the Mass" (Second Vatican Council 1963, no. 55).

The reasons why this physical receiving is so highly prized are rich and multiple. They are rooted in the mystery of the incarnation, in which the Godhead was intimately wed to creation through the birth of the Only Begotten. Jesus' own ministry displayed an intimate engagement with flesh and blood folk and the stuff of creation. His table ministry, culminating in the Last Supper, was not an invitation into some kind of gnostic experience but the embodied practice of eating and drinking. This tangible and public act was a continued source of critique and condemnation by his opponents (e.g., Mark 2:16; Matt 9:10; Luke 5:30). According to Henri de Lubac, the table was also the birthplace of the church as, "literally speaking . . . the Eucharist makes the Church" (de Lubac 2006, p. 88). Later theological developments will distinguish this eucharistic presence from other modes of Christ's presence—e.g., in the Word—as a "substantial" presence. Thus, this mode of presence surpasses all others because "through it Christ becomes present whole and entire, God and Man" (Paul VI 1965, no. 39).

Thus, the dilemma: the reception of communion has evolved as a pastoral and theological high point of participation for Roman Catholics at Mass. This is distinct from medieval and post-Tridentine evidence that points to the elevation of the Host after the consecration as the high point.[1] However, the pandemic with its many closures and restrictions has eliminated communion for multitudes of Roman Catholics. While livestreaming the eucharistic liturgy clearly feeds people's spiritualities, it falls short of meeting this need for eucharistic reception.

2. Eucharistic Deprivation and Abstinence: An Historical Perspective

In one sense, the pandemic currently sweeping across the globe and enveloping Christianity in its wake (and thus Roman Catholicism) has created a unique dilemma. Yet, it has some historical precedents. There is clear evidence in the history of Christianity that in different times and places significant numbers of the baptized have been deprived of the eucharist, sometimes because of their own sense of unworthiness. The celebrated bishop and mystagogue John Chrysostom (d. 407) preached powerfully against anyone who was unworthy who dared to receive communion. Not only does he warn against the baptized receiving "this Body into an evil soul", but also cautions clergy against admitting anyone to communion who is known to be unworthy. Both baptized and clergy who engage in such worthiness are, in Chrysostom's estimation, the same as the betrayer

1 Eamon Duffy summarizes this evolution by noting that by this point "for most of the people, most of the time the Host was something to be seen, not to be consumed" (Duffy 2005, p. 95).

Judas (Chrysostom 1986, 82:6). At the same time Chrysostom complained that some folk limited their reception to major feast days, lamenting that even though the "sacrifice is offered", yet no one comes forth for communion (Chrysostom 2002, 3:4).

Multiple factors led to this eventually wide-spread practice of communal and individual withdrawal from the table. One significant element was an evolving self-awareness of the laity that inverted from viewing themselves as the body of Christ to a deeply diminished self-image as a community of sinners and penitents. A burgeoning theology of original sin and the prominent specter of purgatory in the imaginations of the faithful loomed large in this development. While Chrysostom was a voice from the early church that raised concern about declining numbers of communicants, that trend developed so dramatically that the Fourth Lateran Council (1215) had to mandate that people go to communion at least once a year (Mansi 1901–1927, no. 21, 22:1010). Despite this directive the communion of the faithful remained an infrequent event for many baptized. Those belonging to religious communities often needed the permission of their superior or spiritual director to receive, regularly restricted to four or six times a year. In the 17th century the movement known as Jansenism, which strongly emphasized the depravity and corruption of human beings, responded by valuing abstinence from communion and upheld it as a mark of holiness equal to that of actual reception (Mitchell 2009, p. 463).

The so call "plague of Saint Charles" that struck the region of Lombardy from 1575–76, particularly its capital Milan, is an informative episode in this history of eucharistic deprivation. According to his biographer, Milan's Archbishop Charles Borromeo threw himself into the midst of this epidemic, providing both material and spiritual relief to his people (Giussano 1884, pp. 367ff). He not only went among his people distributing communion, but "he directed that every one should hear Mass devoutly each day; and to give effect to this order, he erected altars at the crossways and conspicuous places, where Mass was said daily, so that all could assist from their windows" (Giussano 1884, p. 419). His biographer makes no mention of spiritual communion regarding this (or any other) event, and Borromeo gives scant attention to the topic in his writings. Nonetheless, this unique example of virtual eucharist certainly provided that opportunity for its home-bound participants.

A different sort of eucharistic deprivation became prominent in the so-called age of discovery, when sea-faring European adventurers set out to explore the globe and claim new territories. Roman Catholic missionaries such as the Franciscans and Dominicans ordinarily accompanied Portuguese and Spanish explorers, a trend that both continued and expanded in ensuing centuries. Thus, Stephen Bevans (2002) summarizes: "The modern missionary era was in many ways the 'religious arm' of colonialism, whether Portuguese and Spanish colonialism in the sixteenth Century, or British, French, German, Belgian or American colonialism in the nineteenth". While many missionaries established churches and even compounds in colonial settles, they often ventured beyond those sites to seek converts. This sometimes involved establishing ties with remote villages or outposts that could be revisited to sustain believers. Such visits were generally few and far between. One documentable example in the United States was Fr. Pierre Yeves Kéralum OMI (d. 1872). He was a member of the "Calvary of Christ", a group of Oblate clergy who traveled by horseback throughout the Rio Grande area ministering to far flung Catholics at their ranches and settlements. Three times a year he would make a missionary circuit to some 70 to 120 places spread over a vast territory in the Texas wilderness (Wright n.d.). Between such visits the Catholic families would naturally be deprived Eucharist until the next circuit. This continues to be the situation in many places. My own Capuchin community's ministry in Nicaragua requires our friars to travel by boat or horseback in order to stay in touch with communities they can sometimes visit only once a year.

In the 20th century radio and eventually television emerged as new pastoral tools for reaching believers incapable of being physically present for Mass. One of the earliest examples occurred in Australia when Sydney was chosen as the site for the 1928 Eucharistic Congress. Catholic organizers of the Congress considered it a prime moment for evangelization at a time when over 95% of the Australian population was Christian and almost 25% Roman Catholic (Australian Bureau of Statistics 1921). Consequently, Catholic leadership rented time on the newly established radio station 2UE, first broadcasting special services from Sydney's St. Mary's Cathedral leading up to a live broadcast of the Congress' opening Mass (Griffen-Foley 2008, p. 34).

In the late 1940's Roman Catholic Mass was first broadcast on television, initially on Christmas eve from Paris' Notre Dame Cathedral in 1948. The following year the Christmas Midnight Mass was televised from Boston's Cathedral of the Holy Cross. Such moves were not without controversy. The celebrated German theologian Karl Rahner (d. 1984) strongly objected to televised Mass, arguing that "philistines of the 21st century" should not be allowed to view whatever they wanted while "sitting in an armchair and ... chewing a roll" (Rahner 1953, pp. 182–83). Despite such objections, the number of televised Masses grew rapidly. Already in 1955, the Archdiocese of Boston inaugurated the CatholicTV Network: its first program was a Mass celebrated by the archbishop. This service continues yet today. As such productions multiplied, they were increasingly billed as Masses for "Shut-ins". This evolution acknowledged another group of folks regularly deprived of the Eucharist: the sick or the elder unable to regularly fulfill their Sunday obligation. A Canadian version of "Mass for Shut-ins", first appearing in 1963, is one of the longest running shows in that country's television history (MacDonald 2020). The practice is so widespread in the United States that in 1996 the United States Catholic Conference of Bishops published "Guidelines for Televising the Liturgy" (USCCB 1996).

3. Spiritual Communion as a Roman Catholic Pastoral Response

Obviously, Roman Catholicism is not the only church confronted with this unexpected stricture on the eucharistic table. Most Christian communities are facing this predicament and have mustered a wide range of responses. Some communities have begun the practice of delivering individual packages of consecrated bread and wine to congregants so that they could receive communion during a live streamed broadcast of the church's Sunday worship (Millard and Paulsen 2020). Related is the emerging practice of "drive-thru communion", in which pre-packaged Communion elements are given to folk through their car window, often in the parking lot of an established church (Pine Castle United Methodist Church n.d.). I know of some Roman Catholic communities that provide drive-thru communion following Sunday morning Mass, which draws a larger number of participants that current guidelines allow for face-to-face worship. A more inventive solution has been mailing consecrated elements to folk through via post, particularly in the United States and England. While bishops of some denominations have authorized this activity, others have severely criticized it (Williams 2020).

One of the more widespread and controverted practices is some form of "virtual communion", in which believers assemble appropriate elements from their own households (e.g., crackers or bread and wine or grape juice) and employ them for communion at the appropriate time in the live streamed or replayed rite. This is not a new practice. California's mega-church Saddleback in the Baptist tradition has provided guidelines for this kind of virtual communion since 2014 (Saddleback Church 2014). However, since the onset of the COVID-19 pandemic and the shuttering of churches, this practice has escalated dramatically while igniting widespread debate: often within a single denomination. Internet postings confirm that individual Anglican, Episcopal, Lutheran, Methodist, Presbyterian as well as Evangelical congregations are engaged in this practice.

While multiple denominations have found viable modes for communion in virtual worship, current Roman Catholic magisterial teaching does not recognize the validity of virtual sacraments. The most explicit example of such teaching during the COVID-19 pandemic is a note from the Apostolic Penitentiary (2020) on the Sacrament of Reconciliation, which instructs that even in this pandemic that sacrament is administered in according with universal canon law, i.e., person to person. Previously, the Pontifical Council for Social Communications (2002) emphasized the essential nature of such a "real interpersonal community" as well as "the incarnational reality of the sacraments" (no. 5). It concludes, "Virtual reality is no substitute for the Real Presence of Christ in the Eucharist, the sacramental reality of the other sacraments and shared worship in a flesh-and-blood human community. There are no sacraments on the Internet" (no. 9). Besides the clear prohibition against "virtual communion", this author cannot find any pastoral directives permitting the shipping of consecrated hosts to congregants or dropping them off at homes of the faithful for consumption during live-streamed worship. Such practices fall outside the directives for "Holy Communion outside Mass" found in the 1973 decree by the Sacred Congregation for Divine Worship (1976) "Eucharistic Worship outside Mass". Those directives make it clear that such communion requires an ordinary or extraordinary minister of communion (no. 20). At the same time, these official instructions do not ensure that such practices are absent in Roman Catholic communities.

More accepted and widespread in my tradition is the invitation for on-line worshippers to engage in the practice of spiritual communion at the appropriate time in the rite. Pope Francis has advocated this practice, and on more than one occasion has led the faithful on-line in a traditional prayer for spiritual communion, e.g., on 21 March 2020 using that of Alphonsus Liguori (Mares 2020). Despite this papal example, to some this might yet appear to be a quite inadequate substitute for the "real thing", a kind of pseudo-sacrament in which the priest does not take part because he always gets to receive physical communion. The history and theology of this previously revered practice, however, is infinitely richer and offers a valuable spiritual pathway for believers, and not only in time of pandemic.

A distinction between receiving the eucharistic bread sacramentally and receiving it spiritually stretches all the way back to Augustine (d. 430). In his Tractates on the Gospel of John (Augustine 1988, 26:11–12) the bishop of Hippo instructs the baptized to eat not only on the outside, with one's teeth, but also feast on the inside in one's heart. This is eating the heavenly bread in a spiritual sense. It is not until the Middle Ages, however, that a more developed theology of spiritual communion evolves. In its origins this "mystical approach to the Eucharist", as Gary Macy calls it, was a corrective to a theology of the Eucharist rooted in the teachings of Paschasius Radbertus (1969, d. 865). In Paschasius' pioneering work on the nature of eucharistic presence, *De Corpore et Sanguine Domini*, this 9th century monk was the first theologian to attempt explaining in a systematic and doctrinal way "how" Christ was eucharistically present. In his explanation, Paschasius proposed that the relationship between the historical body and the eucharistic body of Christ was one of identity, not merely continuity (4:1). While understanding that this presence was not just corporeal but also spiritual and mystical, his language and frameworks were insufficient to negotiate these nuances and the fundamental explanation was prone to collapse into physicality. While rejected by theologians such as Thomas Aquinas (d. 1274) and ultimately by the Church's magisterium that took a more metaphysical and sacramental approach, Paschasius' approach was easily and deeply embraced by the faithful and many theologians. In essence, Paschasius taught when we received communion we feasted on the same flesh of Jesus born of Mary, though offered gently and humanely through bread which served as a kind of visual envelope for the Lord's corporeal presence.

It was in response to this inventive yet crude explanation of Christ's eucharistic presence that the more mystical approach emerged. Early formulations distinguished between the sacrament the faithful receive on earth and the heavenly bread on which the angels feed. Although all who receive eucharistic bread on earth do receive the "true" body and blood of Christ, it is only the good who receive the bread of heaven by which one is joined to Christ in faith and love (Macy 1984, p. 76). This soteriological argument rejected any Paschasian claim that feasting on the body of Christ alone was sufficient for salvation: a stance based on a passage in a letter Paschasius wrote to Fredugard, a fellow monk of St-Riquier Monastery. Instead, it (re-) introduced the role of virtue, integrity and spiritual union into the equation of effective and grace-filled communion reception.

Though overshadowed by theologians of the 13th century, Hugh of Saint-Victor (d. 1141) crafted a profound and influential theology of eucharist in this mystical tradition. The abbey of Saint-Victor near Paris followed the Augustinian rule, and Hugh imbibed the Augustinian synthesis that emphasized the union of heaven and earth and the union of the baptized with each other that the eucharist both symbolized and enabled. Gary Macy has well summarized the various strands of Hugh's teaching on the issue of communion and its relationship to salvation (Macy 1984, pp. 83–85). Hugh and those of his school held that the whole of salvation history moves towards spiritual union with Christ. Through the working of the Holy spirit, by the sacraments—especially baptism and Eucharist—people experience the graces of faith and love that lead to this union. According to Hugh, the physical presence of the historical Jesus leads us through his outward appearance to his spiritual existence and, therefore, leads to our mystical union with Christ in faith and love. The eucharist does the same through the use of bread and wine. As Macy summarizes, "this spiritual union in faith and love, toward which all salvation history tends, is by far the most important aspect of the Eucharist for Hugh. To receive the sacrament worthily one must receive in faith and love. Further, if one cannot receive the outward sign of the Eucharist, faith and love alone are sufficient to gain the spiritual union with Christ" (Macy 1984, p. 83).

Other medieval theologians emphasized the centrality of this spiritual reality in their own eucharistic theologies. Some distinguished between reception *corporaliter* and reception *spirtualiter.* This distinction further counters the Paschasian view that weds salvation to the physical consuming of the eucharistized bread. Instead, it emphasizes that simply consuming the bread does not lead one to salvation. It is only by imitating Christ in faith and love and thus participating in the spiritual reception as well does one follow the salvific path (Macy 1984, p. 84). Some authors held that spiritual reception does not require the physical consumption of the sacrament. Apparently, Hugh of St. Victor's own "spiritual communion" on his death bed without sacramental reception—witnessed by the monk Osbert of Clare who later reported it in his correspondence (Macy 1984, p. 95)—confirms the theologian's deep convictions about the primacy of this spiritual union.

Famous mystics of the same period, often through deeply intimate reflections, attested to the efficacy of this form of spiritual union. One of more celebrated examples is that of Mechtild of Magdeburg (Mechtild of Magdeburg 1998, d. about 1282). Her extensive writings document both her deep eucharistic devotion and belief in the power of spiritual communion as well. She was part of a religious movement of women in the 12th and 13th centuries who lived a form of lay religious life in the world. One of the marks of this movement was their practice of receiving communion very frequently, i.e., weekly and sometimes even daily for which they "practically waged war against their confessors and superiors to attain permission" (Macy 1984, p. 90). Despite this increased frequency, Mechtild yet pens a spiritual complaint turned revelation "that she hears no Mass nor Hours and How God Praises her in ten things".

I who am Divine am truly in you.

I can never be sundered from you:

However far we be parted,

never can we be separated.

I am in you and you are in Me.

We could not be any closer.

We two are fused into one,

poured into a single mould.

Thus, unwearied,

we shall remain

forever.

(Mechtild, p. 111)

This intense expression of mystical communion epitomizes a trend in which spiritual communion was theologically affirmed, pastorally promoted and personally cherished.

The insertion of the elevation of the bread into the eucharistic liturgy, already in some places by the end of the 12th century, provided a new opportunity for practicing spiritual communion during the Mass. One caution, however, is that we do not have clear evidence when exactly people engaged in this practice. Works like the 13th century *Ancrene Wisse* (Hasenfrantz 2000) note that "salutations" were to be recited during the elevation (e.g., "Hail, provision on our pilgrimage"). Some of these were repeated in the 14th century *The Lay Folks Mass Book*. (Simons [1879] 2008) There is a difference between "adoration" and "spiritual communion". The saluting of the host was clearly an act of adoration. It is not clear, however, how often such engagement was intentional spiritual communion properly understood. The same could also be said about the opportunities offered by the burgeoning practice of eucharistic processions.

The virtuous instincts of Hugh of St. Victor for connecting the act of physical reception of communion with the proper spiritual disposition affirmed by an integrity that expressed itself in a faith manifest in love was often overlooked in the ensuing centuries. Some theologians and clergy were concerned that frequent communion could breed indifference to the sacrament. Consequently, preachers often emphasized that spiritual communion brought all of the benefits but none of the risks of actual communion. Dutch theologian Wessel Gansfort (d. 1489) "went so far to argue that spiritual communion was superior to sacramental communion because it was not restricted to specific times, places or persons" (Burnett 2011, p. 84). This extreme view found resonance in the influential teaching and practices of the monastery of Port-Royal in Paris. Aligned with the teachings of Jansenism that emphasized the basic depravity and corruption of all people, the abbess Mere Angélique Arnauld (d. 1661) promoted voluntary abstinence from Communion, claiming that such could be a mark of holiness equal to that of actual reception (Mitchell 2009, p. 463).

4. Healing the Rift

The theological views of Gansfort, Arnauld and others as well as the practices they promoted created an unwelcome divide between reception *corporaliter* and reception *spiritualiter*. Hugh of St. Victor and others of his school understood spiritual reception as an essential part of the physical act of receiving communion worthily. Contrary to a strand of teaching found in the work of Paschasius and his many followers, they taught that consuming the host was insufficient for the heavenly union that the sacrament symbolizes. Instead, intention and desire wed to a life of faith and love were the paths that properly opened the graces of communion. Rather than viewing reception *corporaliter* and *spiritualiter* as both complementary and intrinsically related, however, in practice these became separated realities: the first reserved for the worthy and shriven and the second relegated to the undeserving who avoided physical reception and its threat of damnation if received unworthily. Consequently, even in the present day of frequent communion by Roman Catholics this mystical and deeply spiritual aspect of reception is widely underplayed. Thus, the connection between receiving communion and living a eucharistic life has receded from the consciousness of many a communicant. In this environment, rather than an essential component of eucharistic integrity, spiritual communion can appear to be a pious, vaguely wistful yet ultimately unfulfilling exercise in the absence of "real" reception.

While the COVID-19 pandemic has been an appalling experience on so many levels, that does not preclude it as a context for wisdom both ancient and new. The invitation to spiritual communion—sundered from physical reception for so many who regularly live-stream Mass during this health crisis—is yet an opportunity for catechizing folk about the sacramental reality of desire, the truth of mystical communion, and the multiple modes of Christ's real presence that the Roman Catholic Church acknowledges. As to the former, Christians from the time of Augustine (d. 430) to the present day have affirmed that authentically desiring baptism when it is not physically possible to undergo the ritual is true baptism. In his writings against the Donatists, Augustine holds that baptism can occur through suffering but also by "conversion of heart" (Augustine 1887, 4:22) or what came to be known as baptism of desire. The validity of such baptism was reiterated by Thomas Aquinas (d. 1274) in his *Summa Theologica* (e.g., Aquinas 1947, III, q. 68, art. 2), upheld by Alphonsus Liguori (de Liguori 1852, Bk 6, II, 1, 96), confirmed in the Catechism of Pius X (2015, p. 65), and is further recognized by the current *Catechism of the Catholic Church* (1992, no. 1258).

Similarly, mystics and theologians have affirmed in their teachings and personal practices that desiring Eucharist is not simply a pious exercise but also a doctrinally affirmed, real encounter with the eucharistic Christ (Costa 2012, p. 139). Aquinas himself argues that while it is not equal to the full experience of sacramental communion, spiritual communion—or communion *in voto*—is nonetheless an effective and grace filled activity (Aquinas 1947, III, q. 80, a. 1, ad 3). In two different sessions, the Council of Trent also recognized the validity and importance of spiritual Communion (Session 13, chp. 8; Session 22, chp. 6). In other words, spiritual communion is "real" communion, although not as perfect as physical reception. Due to the Roman Catholic insistence on Christ's real presence in the consecrated species, "real presence" has been a phrase unfortunately confined to the eucharistized elements. However, the Constitution on the Sacred Liturgy from Vatican II—largely drawing on the teaching of Pius XII's encyclical *Mediator Dei* (1947)—authoritatively taught that Christ is present in five different ways: (1) in the person of the minster, (2) under the eucharistic species, (3) in the sacraments, (4) in the Word, and (5) in the assembly (Second Vatican Council 1963, no. 7). This is a teaching yet to settle deeply into the spiritualities of most Roman Catholics, who are inclined to posit "real presence" only of the consecrated elements. The other 4 modes of that presence are perceived—if at all—as shadows of the one "true" presence under the appearances of bread and wine.

The Christological reality, however, is that Christ never promises to be partially present. Thus, Christ's presence in the proclamation of the gospel is not a 60% rendering of the presence of the eternal Logos. Nor is the assembly some tarnished reflection of the Body of Christ. On the contrary, long before there were tabernacles or reserved sacraments or eucharistic devotion, Paul was asserting that the community is the Body of Christ (1 Cor. 12:27). This expansive Christological rethinking find its most jarring expression in the often-overlooked assertion of Christ's presence in the sacraments, i.e., when anyone baptizes "it is really Christ who baptizes" (Second Vatican Council 1963, no. 7). This means that when a Jewish or Muslim nurse working in a neonatal unit, surrounded by days old infants, discerns that one of the newborns identified as "Catholic" is in danger of death and then baptizes, Christ is present: this despite the fact that there may not be a single Christian in the room.

Real presence in this expansive sense is a recovered yet often unexplored gift of conciliar and post-conciliar theology. When quarantined folk join a live-streamed eucharist and listen to the Word proclaimed, they experience the true presence of Christ. The power of God's Word does not evaporate over the Internet. Similarly, digital broadcasts do not impede experiencing presiders or even other baptized as they populate a zoom or Facebook worship space as authentic encounters with the Lord's presence. Different—definitely! Inauthentic—no! Therefore, too, communing spiritually with the presider through televised Mass is true communing, albeit not its fullest expression.

Advances in media theory and theological reflections on emerging understandings of issues such as virtual presence and digital communities bolster this position. Already in 1998, the Roman Catholic theologian Tom Beaudoin was exploring video games, MTV videos, music and cyberspace as venues where generation X was forging its own theologies. In Beaudoin's language, this allowed alternative ways of being virtually religious, and even engaging in virtual liturgy. In a visionary way, Beaudoin recognized that "cyberspace" held the potential for virtual communities where virtual religion could be practiced (Beaudoin 1998, pp. 37–49). With the expansion of the world wide web, especially in the early 21st century, theorizing about virtual presence, online religion and digital communities blossomed. Margaret Wertheim was a pioneering voice, arguing that the very essence of cyberspace is its capacity to service as a network of relationships and a technologically realized new heaven (Wertheim 1999, esp. 120–54). In shaping methodologies for studying religion in cyberspace Christopher Helland proposed a widely employed distinction between online religion and religion online. The former characterizes websites that encourage the interactivity of web users, while the latter were more content driven with little or no possibilities for interaction (Helland 2000). It was the former, he argued, that were important for the shaping of community. While this binary framework has been criticized for its lack of porosity (Young 2004), it nonetheless shows the continuing quest for discovering how cyberspace supports and encourages communitas. Similarly, non-religious works dating back to Howard Rheingold's ([1993] 2000) *The Virtual Community*, have argued for both the real possibility and definite value of this digital fellowship while also recognizing its limitations and shadow sides.

The contributions from media theory take a particular turn and confront questions they cannot answer alone, however, when it comes to sacramental worship. As Heidi Campbell recognizes, it is one thing to speak about the internet as a medium for facilitating spiritual experiences, or a tool for promoting religion, or as a technology for affirming the religious life and traditions of a community. It is another to consider it a "sacramental space" (Campbell 2005, p. 11). This has particular ramifications for Roman Catholic eucharistic theology, which is not always properly understood by contemporary commentators on virtual worship.[2] Teresa Berger, the Thomas E. Golden Professor of Catholic Theology at Yale, provides a useful context for pondering such questions by underscoring that Christian worship itself has always been "mediated", and that digital technologies stand in a long line of liturgical mediations (Berger 2018, pp. 7–8). She also smartly recognizes that digitally mediated worship is not disembodied but entails its own specific bodily proprieties (Berger 2018, p. 20). Finally, she illustrates that an ecclesial community beyond spatial proximity is possible and that Church cannot be simply defined by the physical co-presence of believers (Berger 2018, p. 44). On the other hand, Berger acknowledges that the most challenging issuing here concerns questions of sacramental practices in digital mediation (Berger 2018, p. 75). When it comes to eucharist she does not advocate for digitally mediated eucharistic sharing (Berger 2018, p. 96). She does recognize, however, that our rich traditional of sacramentality provides a context for recognizing virtual eucharist as broadly "sacramental". This is not, however, the same as receiving the consecrated elements that Roman Catholics believe mediate a unique and substantial presence of Christ (see Labenek 2014, esp. 42–50). Thus, spiritual communion as a digitally mediated encounter, in the context of an on-line ecclesial event, framed by Christ's presence in the Word, is rightly understood as a sacramental exercise—though not properly understood as a sacrament. Paradoxically, physically receiving communion is itself an experience of presence and absence (Parish 2020), i.e., an absence of the historical body of Christ, one of the three bodies of Christ recognizes by ancient church teaching

5. Conclusions

Nathan Mitchell has insightfully recognized that the emergence of sacraments of desire, including spiritual communion, were valid attempts to broaden access to sacraments "without denying the legitimacy or necessity of the Church's liturgical celebrations" (Mitchell 2009, p. 463). One could argue in that same vein that eucharistic forays into the

[2] Daniel Bare, for examples, misunderstands the Roman Catholic teaching about transubstantiation as he contends "The Roman Catholic Church holds that the bread and wine transubstantiate, that their substance is transformed into the literal, physical body and blood of Christ." (Bare 2020, 37) Bare fails to recognize that substance is a metaphysical not physical construct, and cannot be changed into the physical body and blood of Christ. The Roman Catholic Church holds for a true, real and substantial presence but one present in a sacramental and not physical mode.

media—be that radio, television, or the Internet—are valid contemporary endeavors for achieving that same access while simultaneously affirming the central import of that key ecclesial ritual, Sunday Mass.

Spiritual communion has reemerged in Roman Catholic consciousness as an appropriate, even necessary form of the active participation mandated by the Constitution on the Sacred Liturgy (no. 14). Unfortunately, this under catechized and little theologized practice yet suffers under the veil of a kind of sour grapes spirituality, i.e., it is the best we can do, although it leaves a bad taste in our mouths. While I long for the return to a nave overflowing with the baptized, full throated singing without masks, and communion lines replete with "Amens" that echo after each moment of sharing bread and cup, I also long for a renewed commitment to spiritual communion. This is a yearning for a deep consciousness among communicants—including the clergy—that authentic reception is not simply *corporaliter* but also *spiritualiter*. It is only in reuniting these too often severed perspectives that we can fulfill Augustine's challenge, and become what we eat (Augustine 1997, Sermon 272).

Funding: This research received no external funding.

Institutional Review Board Statement: Not applicable.

Informed Consent Statement: Not applicable.

Conflicts of Interest: The author declares no conflict of interest.

References

Apostolic Penitentiary. 2020. Note from the Apostolic Penitentiary on the Sacrament of Reconciliation in the Current Pandemic. March 20. Available online: https://press.vatican.va/content/salastampa/en/bollettino/pubblico/2020/03/20/200320d.html (accessed on 8 March 2021).

Aquinas, Thomas. 1947. *The Summa Theologia*. Translated by Fathers of the English Dominican Province. New York: Benziger Brothers.

Augustine. 1887. *Baptism, Against the Donatists*. Translated by J. R. King. New York: Charles Scribner's Sons.

Augustine. 1988. *Tractates on the Gospel of John 11–27*. The Fathers of the Church, 79. Translated by John Rettig. Washington, DC: Catholic University of America Press.

Augustine. 1997. "Sermon 272". Trans. Nathan Mitchell. *Assembly* 23: 14.

Australian Bureau of Statistics. 1921. Census of the Commonwealth of Australia. Available online: https://www.ausstats.abs.gov.au/ausstats/free.nsf/0/F71203E9C651751CCA2578390015AB47/$File/1921%20Census%20-%20Volume%20I%20-%20Part%20VI%20Religions.pdf (accessed on 8 March 2021).

Bare, Daniel. 2020. How Embodied is 'the Body of Christ?' COVID-19 and Christian Corporeality. In *Religion in Quarantine: The Future of Religion in a Post-Pandemic World*. Edited by Heidi Campell. pp. 36–38. Available online: https://oaktrust.library.tamu.edu/bitstream/handle/1969.1/188004/Religion%20in%20Quarantine-PDF-eBook-final-2020.pdf?sequence=4&isAllowed=y (accessed on 8 March 2021).

Beaudoin, Tom. 1998. *Virtual Faith: The Irreverent Spiritual Question of Generation X*. San Francisco: Jossey-Bass.

Berger, Teresa. 2018. *@ Worship: Liturgical Practices in Digital Worlds*. New York: Routledge.

Bevans, Stephen. 2002. New Evangelical Vision and Mission. *Divine Word Missionary Magazine*.

Burnett, Amy Nelson. 2011. The Social History of communion and the Reformation of the Eucharist. *Past & Present* 211: 77–119.

Campbell, Heidi. 2005. Spiritualising the internet. Uncovering discourses and narratives of religious internet usage. *Online. Heidelberg Journal of Religions on the Internet* 1: 1–26.

Catechism of the Catholic Church. 1992. Available online: https://www.vatican.va/archive/ENG0015/_INDEX.HTM (accessed on 8 March 2021).

Chrysostom, John. 1986. *Homilies on the Gospel of St. Matthew*, Rev. ed. Nicene and Post-Nicene Fathers. Translated by George Prevost. Grand Rapids: Eerdmans, vol. 10.

Chrysostom, John. 2002. *Homilies on Galatians, Ephesians, Philippians, Colossians, Thessalonians, Timothy, Titus, and Philemon*. Nicene and Post-Nicene Fathers. Grand Rapids: Eerdmans, vol. 13.

Code of Canon Law. 1983. Available online: http://www.vatican.va/archive/cod-iuris-canonici/cic_index_en.html (accessed on 8 March 2021).

Costa, Francis. 2012. Nature and Effects of Spiritual Communion. *Proceedings of the Catholic Theological Society of America* 13: 139–47.

de Liguori, Alphonsus. 1852. *Theologia Moralis*. Edited by Michael Heilig. Mechlin: P.J. Hanicq, vol. 6.

de Lubac, Henri. 2006. *Corpus Mysticum: The Eucharist and the Church in the Middle Ages*. Translated by Gemma Simmonds. Edited by Laurence Paul Hemming and Susan Frank Parsons. Notre Dame: University of Notre Dame Press.

Duffy, Eamon. 2005. *The Stripping of the Altars: Traditional Religion in England, 1400–1450*, 2nd ed. New Haven and London: Yale University Press.

Gambino, Mathew. 2019. Half of Catholics Attending Mass 28 Years Ago no Longer Do, Figures Show. September 5. Available online: CatholicPhilly.com (accessed on 8 March 2021).

Giussano, John Peter. 1884. *The Life of St. Charles Borromeo*. London: Burnes and Oates.

Griffen-Foley, Bridget. 2008. Radio Ministries: Religion on Australian Commercial Radio from the 1920s to the 1960s. *Journey of Religious History* 32: 31–53. [CrossRef]

Hasenfrantz, Robert, ed. 2000. *Ancrene Wisse*. Kalamazoo: Medieval Institute Publications.

Helland, Christopher. 2000. Religion Online/Online Religion and Virtual communitas. In *Religion on the Internet: Research Prospects and Promises*. Edited by Jeffery Hadden and Douglas Cowan. London: Jai Press/Elsevier Science, pp. 205–24.

Labenek, Andrew. 2014. The Promise and Problematic of the Virtual Eucharist Mass According to the Roman Catholic Church's Position in 'The Church and the Internet'. Master's thesis, University of Western Ontario, London, ON, Canada. Available online: https://ir.lib.uwo.ca/cgi/viewcontent.cgi?article=3306&context=etd (accessed on 8 March 2021).

Macy, Gary. 1984. *The Theologies of the Eucharist in the Early Scholastic Period*. Oxford: Clarendon Press.

Mansi, Giovanni Domenico. 1901–1927. *Sacrorum Conciliorum Nova et Amplissima Collectio*. Paris: H. Welter.

Mares, Courtney. 2020. Pope Francis Offers this Spiritual Communion Prayer during Coronavirus Pandemic. *Catholic News Agency*. March 21. Available online: https://www.catholicnewsagency.com/news/pope-francis-offers-this-spiritual-communion-prayer-during-coronavirus-pandemic-53326 (accessed on 8 March 2021).

MacDonald, Ryan. 2020. COVID-19: As Churches Close, Many Turn to 'Mass for Shut-ins' Service. Available online: https://atlantic.ctvnews.ca/covid-19-as-churches-close-many-turn-to-mass-for-shut-ins-service-1.4860822 (accessed on 8 March 2021).

Mechtild of Magdeburg. 1998. *The Flowing Light of the Godhead*. The Classics of Western Spirituality. Translated by Frank Tobin. New York and Mahwah: Paulist Press.

Millard, Egan, and David Paulsen. 2020. Drive Through Communion? Remote Consecration? COVID-19 Sparks Eucharistic Experimentation—And Theological Debate. *Episcopal News Service*. April 8. Available online: https://www.episcopalnewsservice.org/2020/04/08/drive-thru-communion-remote-consecration-covid-19-sparks-new-eucharistic-concepts-and-theological-questions/ (accessed on 8 March 2021).

Mitchell, Nathan. 2009. Eucharist Adoration Revisited. *Worship* 83: 457–71.

Old St. Patrick's Church. n.d. Available online: https://livestream.com/oldstpats/events/4667723 (accessed on 8 March 2021).

Parish, Helen. 2020. The Absence of Presence and the Presence of Absence: Social Distancing, Sacraments, and the Virtual Religious community during the COVID-19 Pandemic. *Religions* 11: 276. [CrossRef]

Paul VI. 1965. Mysterium Fidei. Available online: http://www.vatican.va/content/paul-vi/en/encyclicals/documents/hf_p-vi_enc_03091965_mysterium.html (accessed on 8 March 2021).

Pine Castle United Methodist Church. n.d. Drive-Thru Communion. Available online: https://pinecastleumc.com/drive-through-communion (accessed on 8 March 2021).

Pius X, Pope. 1910. Quam Singulari. Available online: https://www.papalencyclicals.net/pius10/p10quam.htm (accessed on 8 March 2021).

Pius X, Pope. 2015. *Catechism of Saint Pius X*. London: Aeterna Press.

Pius XII, Pope. 1953. Christus Dominus. Available online: https://www.papalencyclicals.net/pius12/p12chdom.htm (accessed on 8 March 2021).

Pius XII, Pope. 1957. Sacram Communionem. Available online: https://www.papalencyclicals.net/pius12/p12fast.htm (accessed on 8 March 2021).

Pontifical Council for Social Communications. 2002. The Church and Internet. February 22. Available online: http://www.vatican.va/roman_curia/pontifical_councils/pccs/documents/rc_pc_pccs_doc_20020228_church-internet_en.html# (accessed on 8 March 2021).

Radbertus, Paschasius. 1969. *De corpore et sanguine Domini: Cum appendice Epistola ad Fredugardum*. Corpus Christianorum Continuatio Mediaevalis 16. Edited by Peda Paulus. Turnholt: Brepols.

Rahner, Karl. 1953. Die Messe und das Fernsehen. *Orientierung* 7: 179–83.

Rheingold, Howard. 2000. *The Virtual Community*, 2nd ed. Cambridge: MIT Press. First Published 1993.

Sacred Congregation for Divine Worship. 1976. Eucharistic Worship outside Mass. In *The Rites of the Catholic Church*. New York: Pueblo Publishing, vol. 1, pp. 447–512.

Saddleback Church. 2014. Take Communion Online with Us. 24.i. Available online: https://saddleback.com/archive/blog/internet-campus/2014/01/24/take-communion-online-with-us (accessed on 8 March 2021).

Second Vatican Council. 1963. Sacrosanctum Concilium. Available online: https://www.vatican.va/archive/hist_councils/ii_vatican_council/documents/vat-ii_const_19631204_sacrosanctum-concilium_en.html (accessed on 8 March 2021).

Simons, Thomas Frederick. 2008. *The Lay Folks' Mass Book: Or the Manner of Hearing Mass, with Rubrics and Devotions for the People*. Whitefish: Kessinger. First Published 1879.

USCCB. 1996. Guidelines for Televised Mass. Available online: https://www.usccb.org/prayer-and-worship/the-mass/frequently-asked-questions/guidelines-for-televising-the-liturgy (accessed on 8 March 2021).

Wertheim, Margaret. 1999. *The Pearly Gates of Cyberspace: A History of Space from Dante to the Internet*. London: Virago Press.

Williams, Hattie. 2020. Holy Communion by Mail 'Non Canonical'. *Church Times*. December 15. Available online: https://www.churchtimes.co.uk/articles/2020/18-december/news/uk/communion-by-mail-pushes-the-envelope-too-far-says-bishop (accessed on 8 March 2021).

Wright, Robert. n.d. Kéralum, Pierre Yeves. Available online: https://www.omiworld.org/lemma/keralum-pierre-yves/ (accessed on 8 March 2021).

Young, Glenn. 2004. Reading and Praying Online: The continuity of Religion Online and Online Religion in Internet Christianity. In *Religion Online: Finding Faith on the Internet*. Edited by Lorne Dawson and Douglas Cowan. New York: Routledge, pp. 93–106.

religions

MDPI

Article

Worship for People with Cognitive Challenges in the Pandemic Era: A Korean Presbyterian Perspective

Hwarang Moon

Korea Theological Seminary, Cheonan 31071, Korea; blauw100@daum.net

Abstract: During COVID-19, many people in the world experienced tremendous suffering. Because of its strong infection rate, people avoided gathering. In these circumstances, public worship, which is the heartbeat of the church, has declined. The decline in participation is especially true among one group of marginalized people: the people who are cognitively challenged. Traditionally, the Korean Church has not had much concern about the matter of public worship and the sacraments for those who are cognitively challenged, except for a few churches which have special departments for ministries to special populations. During the COVID-19 situation, these ministries have slowed, which means that those who benefited have had few opportunities to join worship services or participate in religious education. Going forward, there is a high possibility of another pandemic. Therefore, it is time to prepare for the future. Some churches have utilized online worship and Zoom meetings, showing that the cognitively challenged can effectively participate in online worship and religious education if family members can help them. Churches should invest in new platforms which harmonize onsite worship and online worship and expand resources to create new software for Christian education.

Keywords: cognitively challenged; COVID-19; online worship; participation; church education; Korean Church

1. Introduction

The world is still groaning from the suffering caused by the COVID-19 pandemic. Over the last year, many people have died, and many, despite having recovered, are battling the lasting side effects of the disease. The coronavirus strain, often referenced by its abbreviation, COVID-19, is one of the most highly infectious diseases in history. Health and government officials, in response to the contagious nature of the virus, sought a restricted social atmosphere in order to limit face-to-face contact. Due to health risks associate with meeting or working in groups, social distancing has been implemented according to government regulations in many countries across the globe (Harari 2020).

After many countries reported COVID-19 cases, trade among nations was disrupted, which resulted in a global economic recession. Even though each national government issued some form of aid to its citizens in the form of direct payments to people and financial support to businesses, the financial stability of ordinary people was diminished by shrinking job markets. Unemployment remains high, and it is challenging for those without work to find new jobs.

Churches throughout the world are also facing challenges. After the outbreak of COVID-19 in January 2020, many Korean Churches tried to congregate responsibly while cooperating with the Korean government's guidelines. Even though some churches had incidences of contagion, in general, Korean churches reduced their public gatherings according to social distancing policies.

Many churches chose to offer online worship as an alternative to in-person worship, while other churches recommended family worship while providing guidelines and manuals for in-home worship. These were thought to be "temporary measures," but as time goes on, these measures are still being used. Many pastors and congregations are feeling a greater and greater loss because public worship has traditionally served as the heartbeat of the church. Over the last year in the Korean Church, scholars and laymen alike contemplated and debated such questions as: "Should believers worship together indoors?", "Can online worship be an alternative to public worship?", "Should Christians worship only on Sundays?", "Is an online Eucharist valid?", and "Is it a government responsibility to set restrictions for the number of participants who can safely gather in worship?"[1]

Church leaders are responsibly and thoughtfully addressing the many social, theological, and health concerns that the global pandemic has thrust upon our congregations, but the best interests of members with cognitive disabilities are often overlooked. Traditionally, the Korean Church has not focused a great deal of concern on the matter of worship and sacrament for the cognitively challenged (Moon 2015, pp. 116–20). According to statistics, in the Korean Protestant Church, just about the 400 churches have a special department that focuses on issues concerning worship and the cognitively challenged.[2] The percentage of the population to report cognitive disabilities currently stands at about three percent of the whole population.[3] Despite the statistics on the general population, it is difficult to know the exact percentage of Korean Church congregants with cognitively challenged and which of them regularly participate in worship.

Under the current conditions imposed by the social effects of the coronavirus, the communal worship practices and spiritual support for the cognitively challenged and their families has deteriorated. Some megachurches in Korea broadcast or share recorded video files of sermons for use by those that have mental handicaps, but almost all smaller churches, which compose the majority of the Korean Church, do not have the necessary additional resources to allow for broadcasting or media-sharing.

Even though the vaccine has been developed and the outlook for 2021 looks better, the situation that the pandemic has created could linger or be repeated with a new virus at any time and, therefore, it is necessary to be pro-active. Now is the time to discuss and assess the spiritual needs and worship methods to best serve those parishioners that have cognitive challenges.

2. The Korean Presbyterian Church's Theological Approaches to the Cognitively Challenged

It is necessary to study how Korean Presbyterian churches understand this kind of impairment theologically before arguing the matter of worship and sacrament for the cognitively challenged because theology and practice are closely intertwined.

There are various theological approaches to the cognitively challenged. Some understand it as God's punishment related to human sin; some consider it as an opportunity for healing; others consider it as participation in the suffering of Christ. However, the character of Korean Presbyterian theology can be portrayed as indifference. It is very hard to find cognitively challenged people in the local church. This is reflected in the general lack of resources directed to encouraging and enabling participation of persons who are cognitively challenged. It is very hard to find a denominational document which addresses worship matters and sacraments for cognitively challenged, except two Presbyterian denominations (Tonghap and Kosin).

The Tonghap Church published the denominational document "Guidelines for Baptism of the Mentally Handicapped" in 2005. In their liturgical book, they added some guidelines and liturgy for the inclusion of cognitively challenged people (Korean Presbyterian Church (Tonghap) (2008)). In addition, they open the possibility of inclusion of those who are cognitively challenged in the eucharistic celebrations. Because they had a close relationship with the PCUSA (Presbyterian Church in the USA), they learned and borrowed their theological and practical stance from them.

In case of the Kosin Church, one of the most conservative Protestant churches in Korea, a denominational report on baptism and liturgy for cognitively challenged was written in 2019. They permitted the practice of baptism for the cognitively challenged but do not permit their participation in the Lord's Supper, because they believe that baptism and the Lord's Supper are distinct sacraments. Many believe that baptism and the Lord's Supper require the cognitive ability and faithful confession that the cognitively challenged cannot satisfy. This demonstrates a theological stance of many Korean Churches that diminishes the personhood of cognitively challenged people.

However, liturgical theologian Hwarang Moon's two books *Engraved upon the Heart* (Moon 2015) and *Mapping the Christin Worship* (Moon 2020) impacted the Korean people and enhanced their understanding about worship and sacraments for cognitively challenged people. Based on liturgical theology and religious education, he shows how liturgy impacts faith formation. According to him, it is very important for cognitively challenged people to participate in community worship and sacrament because they learn from participation and practice. While participating in liturgical celebration and sacrament, tacit knowledge is engraved upon the heart and the body (Polanyi and Prosch 1975). Even though they cannot articulate their faith logically, however, something happens in their brain (Polanyi 1967).

At the same time, such persons bring several gifts to other members of the church. Their participation makes real intergenerational worship possible. Each person learns from each other, and all congregants experience new and real friendships, despite differences in age, intelligence, or social status (Swinton 2000, p. 44). While worshipping together, people experience a nurturing of the spirituality and virtue of those who serve. Moreover, it completes the community. While having fellowship, the communal aspect of the church is visible and shows that faith is not merely a personal issue. Stanley Hauerwas says, "Mentally handicapped people are reminders that belief and faith are not individual matters, but faith names the stance of the church as a political body in relation to the world. We are not members of a church because we know what we believe, but we are members of a church because we need the whole church to believe for us (Hauerwas 1994, p. 184). Therefore, in public worship, the presence of the cognitively challenged are needed. By their presence, people can remember who we are and that we are not sufficient but for God's grace (Wadell 1994, pp. 62–63).

3. Analyzing the Current Situation

The following case studies are representative examples of attitudes and practices found among Korean Churches in their approach to worship with and for people with cognitive disabilities during the COVID-19 pandemic.[4] Each case study represents a type or composite of like-minded congregations and is not intended to portray any one congregation.

<Case 1>

Church Type A is a mid-sized church of under 200 congregants. Due to the coronavirus pandemic and in accordance with the Korean Government's policy on social distancing, Church A abruptly organized an online worship for Sunday's public worship. However, they were very busy producing and broadcasting online worship only for Sunday public worship. Because of a lack of labor force and resources, the church does not have any additional resources for preparing the online worship for Sunday school, senior citizens, or those who are cognitively challenged. Sometimes, social distancing protocols were alleviated according to the lower severity of the infection rates, and Church A had a chance to offer onsite worship; however, because of a higher risk of infection for those with disabilities and those over the age of 65, some members were not able to participate in-person. Church A did not have the capacity to provide any additional meetings to meet the needs of high risky populations, such as those with cognitive disabilities. The result is that those persons with cognitive challenges and their families must look for services elsewhere, or wait for the end of COVID-19 in order to be included once again in the worshipping life of Church A.

<Case 2>

Church Type B has a designated minister who is responsible for programs to support congregants who have mental handicaps and their families or caregivers. Even though the number of these special-needs members makes up a small percentage of the total church membership, Church B has managed a fruitful program for many years. When COVID-19 disrupted the usual programming, Church B began to broadcast sermons online that were especially designed to engage their mentally handicapped worshippers. They created this type of service to include family members, so everyone could join online worship from home, including the family members with disabilities. The response to this programming from the families that benefitted from this inclusiveness was positive. Parents and family members reported that their children acknowledged the pastor in the monitor and engaged with the worship similar to their previous experience in the church. With the help of parents or family aids, Church B also started a small group meeting for this group via Zoom on weekdays.

<Case 3>

Church Type C, like Type A, responded to the pandemic with online resources that helped to meet the needs for a majority of the worshipping community. They were not as fortunate as Type B in having a designated staff person responsible for ministering to people with disabilities, but they did not want to ignore the special needs of their members with disabilities. In consideration of the pandemic and the prohibition of gatherings, Church Type C sought to work alongside family members to create resources that would be spiritually enriching for those with disabilities. This approach involved curating a virtual library of shared resources from several different sources. The use of shared resources required that parents or other caregivers be willing to take on the role of a minister for their children with disabilities. Each week volunteers from the church sent links to a curated list of movie clips, picture resources, and/or Sunday School curricula produced by pastors. It was also useful to consult with the "Korea Research Center for Disability ministry" on weekdays. Parents or other relatives would then assume the role of pastor or teacher for their kids using these shared resources. Realizing that parents may be challenged by the responsibility of teaching their kids, the pastors committed to regularly checking in with each parent and answered questions that came up week to week.

There are various other circumstances and solutions than the ones described in the three imagined scenarios listed above; however, these three case studies are representative of the most common responses to the ministry needs of people with cognitive disabilities in the Korean Churches during the pandemic. It is very shocking to learn how few resources are available for the cognitively challenged and their families in the Korean Church during the pandemic, even though they experienced great revival and growth in the world of Christianity prior to the lockdown. This shows that the Korean Church has not adequately concerned itself with the most vulnerable and alienated members of society (Moon 2014).

It is very rare to find a church that has a special department or full-time staff person to provide services for the cognitively challenged in the Korean Church. The pandemic exacerbated an already bad situation, so the cognitively challenged and their families experienced a very difficult time. Because of the danger of infection, all church members severely restricted the level of activity outside of their homes and they developed a tendency to remain at home. Before the coronavirus, churchgoers could experience their social and religious community via weekly participation in worship and church life; however, the loss of that regular communion with people deprived many of a reason for being and drained much of the vibrancy of daily life (Zizioulas 2004, p. 18).[5]

Owing to circumstances beyond their control, online worship became an attractive substitution for in person worship. In the Korean Protestant Church, there are serious pros and cons on each side of the argument for online worship. However, in the case of worship for the mentally handicapped, there needs to be greater thoughtfulness in how online worship can be a satisfactory opportunity for inclusion (Grcevich 2020). Based on the three case studies above, let us further consider the theological and practical issues in this matter.

4. Is Online Worship a Crisis or an Opportunity for the Mentally Handicapped?

During the last year, one of the hot issues within the Korean Church was the debate around online worship. Dominating the media and Christian newspaper headlines were questions such as: "Is online worship a legitimate form or worship?", "Is online worship as meaningful to participants as in-person worship?", and "Is it ethical to use online worship?" Some commentators asserted, "Online worship can weaken the sense of community in the church." Before the outbreak of the coronavirus, many Christians were concerned that the Korean Church faced a troubling upward trend in the number of unchurched people in the country. A new trend, however, is as equally bothersome, revealing a consumer-centered worship that allows for believers to pick and choose the church that offers their favorite worship style (Moon et al. 2020).

The pandemic situation opened people's eyes on this: physical spaces and cyber space all belong to God (Berger 2018, p. 44). While participating in online worship, people experience communion with God and spiritual growth (Foley 2021). If online worship is not an impediment to the real presence of God, then spiritual communion is also possible, in that people worship online "without denying the legitimacy or necessity of the church's liturgical celebrations" (Mitchell 2009, p. 463).

In the case of persons with cognitive disabilities, the move to online worship may offer some potential advantages. Prior to the pandemic, the Korean Church had limited programming for those with cognitive disabilities, and there were few congregations equipped to invite members who are cognitively challenged to participate in weekday worship and/or educational programs. The mentally handicapped and their families must wait until Sunday to experience a religious meeting—and that was only after a long search for a church that offers a special worship service to meet their loved one's needs. Some families attempted to replicate the worship experience in their homes, but most found it over-challenging. Even though there are several Christian TV channels in Korea, there have been no programs geared toward persons who are mentally handicapped. Historically, there have been few media outlets or publishers to offer resources that assist families in Christian education or worship experiences that engage those family members with cognitively challenged. The growth of online opportunities for worship and Christian education that has emerged during the pandemic has opened up many more possibilities for people of all ages and abilities to participate in church. People have come to realize that the mentally handicapped can worship at home with the assistance of parents or family members, without needing to wait until Sunday. It has also opened people's eyes to the various worship and educational resources that an online platform can offer.

In those instances where church members have higher cognitive function, the minister or teacher can meet with them via Zoom or a social media platform without the need for assistance or with only limited help from a family member. For those with more serious cognitive impairments, weekday meetings are possible only when parents or family members are available to participate—requiring their greater time and attention. Zoom meetings hold great potential for offering fellowship during weekdays.[6] A platform has arrived that makes possible an everyday quiet time meeting, if only the church can make it available.

Now the fourth industrial revolution is occurring even in the coronavirus era—with the development of virtual reality, augmented reality, and wearable technology. In the future, the church can provide more vivid religious education for mentally handicapped people. A new age that virtually replicates a physical worship space has come.[7]

What seemed like a loss when in-person worship for the mentally handicapped was reduced, may turn out to be a blessing! If churches with a forward way of thinking can develop an online worship platform and educational software, they can create a great opportunity for the mentally handicapped, especially in the areas of worship and education.

It is important, therefore, to evaluate whether online worship has a positive impact on cognitively challenged people. Church leaders may ask these questions:

"What worship activities can those who are cognitively challenged meaningfully engage in an online environment?", "Can they understand the message and concentrate on the speaker?", "Can they show proper response to the contents of worship?", and "Can online worship be spiritually, emotionally, and socially nourishing for them?"

I want to introduce the story of the Seomoon Church, located in Seoul.[8] Seomoon Church has a special department for the cognitively challenged. After the outbreak of the coronavirus in Seoul, worship could not take place in the church, so they started an online worship during that time. The church broadcasted an online worship, and the parents or family members of the cognitively challenged facilitated the at-home worship process. For example, they would turn on the computer or connect the TV monitor. Parents reported their observations of how their children with disabilities participated and responded to the online worship.

In cases of mild cognitive challenges, the children participated in worship via the online platform in ways that closely resemble their participation during any other form of Sunday worship. They clearly illustrated how the online worship mimicked in-person worship with their minister in the monitor leading the same Sunday worship. Participants showed proper responses to the messages and order of worship during online worship.

In the case of those with moderate to severe disabilities, they danced and mimicked the motions, and listened to the sermon during the preaching time. When their parents first saw their children's jumping or dancing, they misunderstood those responses as disinterest in worship; however, as time progressed, they came to interpret these actions as a personal response of praise and worship. Through the parents' reports and observations, it is clear that, if parents and family members help, the cognitively challenged can not only worship, but also engage in various educational activities in the home.

However, in cases of profound cognitive challenges, the situation was different. It was difficult to determine these participants' responses to online worship. For example, they did not seem to notice the appearance of their pastors or teachers when they appeared online. Family members reported that it was hard to determine what their loved ones were feeling or taking away from the experience. However, the worship time with their families was not a totally meaningless time. Even though they could not express their thoughts, their family members could gain an understanding of their religious thoughts and a lightness of their inner mind.[9]

When we analyze the ratio of the cognitively challenged population, mild handicaps account for about 85% of the population (Tylenda et al. 2007, p. 31). Those in the moderate range comprise about 10% of those considered handicapped, and those in the severe range make up 3%, while the percentage of people that fall within the most profound range is 2%. Therefore, online worship itself can offer the opportunity for worship and educational experiences for a vast majority of those that are counted among the cognitively challenged population, with the caveat that many will still require some level of assistance.

4.1. Evaluation of the Theological Position of Conservative Korean Churches against Online Worship

Many scholars in the Korean Presbyterian Church, especially conservative scholars, express a negative stance on the practice of online worship. They insist that online worship is a temporary and expedient remedy to an unavoidable pandemic situation, and it should be abandoned after the threat of the coronavirus and its variants dissipate.[10] This stance is based on the concern that online worship will destroy the communal aspects of church and the importance of public worship will fade (Kim 2020). This narrow definition of worship, however, fails to recognize the large number of people with disabilities who may actually have a greater benefit from online worship than what is possible in person.

Online worship has clear benefits for people with mild cognitive disabilities and for the families who provide their day-to-day care. That is to say, online worship can provide help for worship, education and community for the cognitively challenged.

The Korean Church needs to hear and accept this challenge: "Why has the Korean Church failed to acknowledge the cognitively challenged as full members, and why has the Church permitted public worship and church life to ignore their needs until now?" Even though some churches have offered separate worship for these members, they failed to make accommodations or provide optimal conditions for full participation in public worship of the church.

Even though the pandemic made the world challenging, it has added new perspectives on the matter of education and worship for the cognitively challenged. Online worship, rather than dividing cognitively challenged people from the church community, has introduced greater opportunities for learning and for becoming accustomed to the atmosphere of worship, including singing hymns and songs.[11]

While participating in online worship, the cognitively challenged can join the online public worship with their family. Until now, most of these members worshipped in a segregated or isolated manner, participating in their own worship; however, during the pandemic, they were able to experience intergenerational and inter-ability worship in which whole congregations could join. In the perspective of average people, online worship for the mentally handicapped may be considered less active participation and difficult to assess the engagement with the contents and meaning of worship. However, people do not know what happens in the minds and brains of others. If the Holy Spirit works, in any situation, faith can be grown in their hearts.[12]

Online worship, even though church members are spatially divided, by the simultaneity of time, can give an opportunity of feeling oneness among the congregation (Berger 2018, pp. 37–41). This can express the real sense of community visibly. Christians are scattered all over the world, but the power of the Holy Spirit creates a union of one church. While joining the online worship, all participants receive the same message, and sing the same hymns. By the work of the triune God and omnipresent, believers can experience the oneness in the simultaneity

People can experience liminality not only in the real site, but also in the cyber space (Madge and O'Connort 2005). In other words, Christ is really present not only in on-site worship, but also in online worship (Thompson 2020). This transcends ethnicity, gender, social status, and intelligence: among them, the cognitively challenged join that group confidently as members.[13]

Therefore, online worship for the cognitively challenged is not an area of service for the weak and segregated but can be a visible confessional act for building the essence of the church and a sense of oneness.

4.2. Preparing the Upcoming Pandemic Situation

Finally, in 2021, the coronavirus vaccine became available throughout the world. With additional medicine being produced, it has shed a ray of hope. However, mutations of the coronavirus have been observed throughout the world, so no one can anticipate precisely when this disease will be perfectly controlled. Disease experts predict that even though the COVID-19 virus will be controlled with treatments and vaccines, at any time, a new worldwide pandemic can happen (Stieg 2021). While considering the COVID-19 pandemic, the church should prepare for the possibility of a future pandemic and prepare for alternative ideas for worship accessibility for the cognitively challenged. It is necessary to consider the following things.

First, ecumenical cooperation is necessary. In case of the Korean Presbyterian Church, because of denominational splits, there are many denominations (Ha 2016, pp. 1–8). Even though each denomination has an educational committee and has an educational curriculum, their energy and financial ability are dispersed, so they cannot invest efficiently in online platforms and software. These are money-consuming processes. Therefore, Korean Churches should cooperate in seeking solutions for this large project. Until now, only the Korea Research Center for Disability Ministry has struggled to seek solutions for accommodating the cognitively challenged.[14] However, currently, this institute is suffering from financial problems. Therefore, instead of investing in only one denomination, it would be better if the Korean Research Center for Disability Ministry could share their resources and be supported by more denominations. It is not easy, however, to unify the Korean Presbyterian denominations. For now, considering the situation of the Korean Presbyterian Church, using the existing Korean Researh Center for Disability Ministry would be easiest and most efficent.

Second, in the case of online worship for the cognitively challenged, it is more efficient that their minister appears on screen rather than other preachers come up. In other words, even though a megachurch's online worship may be more accessible for the cognitively challenged, their weekly preacher will be more helpful. Each church needs to set up an online platform and prepare broadcast facilities and resources. If we think from the perspective of the cognitively challenged, when we see and hear their acquaintances in the monitor, they could think, "Ah … this is worship" or "I get to worship … ." If they see unknown people, because of a lack of an existing relationship, they may have greater trouble understanding the message.

Third, churches should consider their education curriculums for the cognitively challenged, because of their average accelerating aging (Lee 2018). Since 2000, Korean society has come to have concerns about the cognitively challenged and improved institutional infrastructure for the handicapped. However, contrary to this trend in Korean society, the ministry for the handicapped in the church has shrunk. When Korean society did not have concerns about the welfare of the handicapped, the church held an important role and non-Christian parents sought the church to provide educational services for their children. However, the situation has changed: it is very hard to evangelize the new believer, and the cognitively challenged in the church have been aging. However, the worship and education programs in churches stay at the Sunday School level. However, in the situation brought about by the pandemic, the Korean Church should renew the curriculum for the cognitively challenged.

Fourth, online worship is most helpful for the mild and moderate (and, perhaps, severe) mental handicap range, but in the case of the profound handicap range, online worship is not an ideal approach. Eventually, in-person worship and physical gathering is very necessary. When this is possible, the church should match their cognitively challenged members with a small group and support fellowship with other believers. In addition, preparing an institutional policy for the cognitively challenged members' worship and learning in the church congregation is more appropriate because the cognitively challenged can learn through fellowship with other people and in the community.[15]

5. Conclusions

From 2020 until now, the entire world has suffered as a result of the COVID-19 outbreak. In churches, this was observed through the loss of public worship, which is the heartbeat of the spiritual life of believers. Throughout the world, the fourth industrial revolution is ongoing, and public education has changed. The development of online education foresaw the change of the existing educational system, and it will affect the worship and educational practices of churches throughout the world.

During the pandemic, the religious life of the cognitively challenged has atrophied. As a result of indifference in the church, people with handicaps have endured a disproportionately difficult time. However, as I showed in this article, online worship and the appearance of online educational programs provide an opportunity for a course correction so that churches can better meet the spiritual and educational needs of all members.

For the future of ministry for the cognitively challenged, many denominations in the Korean Church should cooperate with each other. It is necessary to help each church equip the online broadcasting systems and share the various software platforms developed for this purpose. For example, there exists a church-union association in South Korea. Each denomination's delegates periodically meet and seek to collaborate. They can share fundraising and proceed in making the educational software.

Above all, the most important thing is to provide the educational resources and guidelines for family members of the cognitively challenged. The development of online systems will only be effectively applied when church and family can successfully cooperate.

Funding: This research received no external funding.

Conflicts of Interest: The author declares no conflict of interest.

Notes

1 These questions are similarly addressed in congregations across the USA and in churches of other countries. Regarding this, see (Foley 2021; Cones 2021).

2 http://kmindmall.com/contents/item.view.new.php?it_id=15504644887018 (accessed on 4 March 2021). For the purposes of this article, any reference to "cognitive disabilities," is referencing those persons who might also be described with the terms "mental retardation", "intellectual disability", and "learning disability". Some people misunderstand the difference between intellectual disability and mental disability or illness: the two main characteristics of intellectual disability are limitation of intellect and lack of adaptive behavior. Because "retarded" and "disabled" convey negative images or stereotypes, this paper prefers to use the term "cognitively challenged" to reflect respect for human life and the full personhood of all who live with such challenges.

3 American Psychiatric Association (2000, pp. 43–44) notes that "Among mentally handicapped persons, about 10 percent fall within the moderate range, 3 percent in the severe range, and only 2 percent in the profound rage."

4 For convenience, I will use Type A, Type B, Type C for naming the description of each of these three hypothetical worship settings.

5 Miroslav Volf says, "Just as others, neither can a Christian exist as a Christian before entering into relation with other Christians" (Volf 1998, p. 178).

6 Of course, Zoom meetings are not enough for deep fellowship. However, if VR and wearable machine would be developed such as that depicted in the movie Kingsman, fellowship among the cognitively challenged can be more enhanced.

7 Regarding virtual reality and augmented reality's potential for special education, see Anderson (2019).

8 http://www.seomoon.org/new_home/ (accessed on 11 March 2021).

9 Even though profound range mentally handicapped has religious potential and spiritual ability. See Nouwen (1997, pp. 49–50).

10 https://www.christiandaily.co.kr/news/91801 (accessed on 13 March 2021).

11 Participation and experience can give great learning opportunity for cognitively challenged. See, for example, Webb-Mitchell (2008, pp. 20–22); and Yong (2007, p. 208). While livestreaming the worship feeds people's spiritualities, it enhance the sense of approachness to the worship (Foley 2021, vol. 12, p. 245).

12 Loder (1998, p. 232) says, "The Divine Spirit dramatically and powerfully penetrates and permeates the whole person so that he is consumed by the Divine presence. Regardless of what point in one's life span such a realization may occur, the totality of the life span from birth to death is brought under the power and purposes of God."

13 Liturgical participation is very important for the process of faith formation. Even though mentally handicapped people have a weak cognitive ability, religious understanding cannot be evaluated by oral articulation and logic. Pivarnik (2012, p. 5) says, "Participation in the sacramental-liturgical experience is meant to lead the participant into ever-greater union with the divine. Liturgical participation in the liturgical worship is not merely liturgical celebration, but is centered on the transformation of the human person through grace in the medium of the church in order to bring the individual back to his or her Creator, the source of being."

14 http://www.kmind.net (accessed on 17 March 2021).

15 Mentally handicapped people can learn by the help of their community. So, belonging to community is very important. See, Vygotsky (1978, p. 86). See also Swinton and Mowat (2006, pp. 239–40). People with severe

disabilities can also learn religious concepts. Fulkerson (2007, p. 41) says, "Individuals with severe disabilities communicate (life infants) at the pre-symbolic(perlocutionary) level and can communicate with other people."

References

American Psychiatric Association. 2000. *Diagnostic and Statistical Manual of Mental Disorders*. Arlington: American Psychiatric Association.

Anderson, Ange. 2019. *Virtual Reality, Augmented Reality and Artificial Intelligence in Special Education: A Practical Guide to Supporting Student with Learning Differences*. London: Routledge.

Berger, Teresa. 2018. *@Worship: Liturgical Practices in Digital Worlds*. London: Routledge.

Cones, Bryan. 2021. Essential Workers, Essential Services? *Leitourgia* in Light of Lockdown. *Religions* 12: 101. [CrossRef]

Foley, Edward. 2021. Spiritual Communion in a Digital Age: A Roman Catholic Dilemma and Tradition. *Religions* 12: 245. [CrossRef]

Fulkerson, Mary McClintock. 2007. *Places of Redemption: Theology for a Worldly Church*. New York: Oxford University Press.

Grcevich, Stephen. 2020. Why Families Think Online Church is Indispensable for Disability Ministry. Available online: https://www.keyministry.org/church4everychild/2020/6/14/why-families-think-online-church-is-indispensable-for-disability-ministry (accessed on 25 July 2021).

Ha, Jaegeon. 2016. Unity and catholicity in the Korean Presbyterian Church: An ecumenical Reformed assessment. *Verbum et Ecclesia* 37: 1–8. [CrossRef]

Harari, Yuval Noah. 2020. The World after Coronavirus. Available online: https://amp.ft.com/content/19d90308-6858-11ea-a3c9-1fe6fedcca75# (accessed on 23 December 2020).

Hauerwas, Stanley M. 1994. The Church and the Mentally Handicapped: A Continuing Challenge to the Imagination. In *Dispatches from the Front: Theological Engagements with the Secular*. Durham: Duke University Press, pp. 177–86.

Kim, Byunghoon. 2020. Online Worship is not Perpect Public Worship. *Kukmin USA*. September 9. Available online: http://ny.kukminusa.com/news/view.php?gisa_id=2020090920275525 (accessed on 14 July 2021).

Korean Presbyterian Church (Tonghap). 2008. *Directory of Worship*. Seoul: Korean Presbyterian Publisher.

Lee, SunHwa. 2018. Measures Should Be Prepared for Middle-Aged and Elderly People with Developmental Disabilities. *Social Focus*. August 20. Available online: https://www.socialfocus.co.kr/news/articleView.html?idxno=235 (accessed on 13 July 2021).

Loder, James E. 1998. *The Logic of the Spirit: Human Development in Theological Perspective*. San Francisco: Jossey-Bass.

Madge, Clare, and Henrietta O'Connort. 2005. Mothers in the Making? Exploring Liminality in Cyber/Space. *Transactions of the Institute of British Geographers* 30: 83–97. [CrossRef]

Mitchell, Nathan. 2009. Eucharist Adoration Revisited. *Worship* 83: 457–71.

Moon, Hwarang. 2014. Including the Mentally Handicapped in Religious Ceremony: Michael Polanyi's Tacit Dimension and Pierre Bouridieu's Habitus. *The Journal of Asian American Theological Forum (AATF)* 1: 31–32.

Moon, Hwarang. 2015. *Engraved upon the Heart: Children, the Cognitively Challenged, and Liturgy's Influence on Faith Formation*. Eugene: Wipf and Stock Publisher.

Moon, Hwarang. 2020. *Mapping the Christian Worship*. Seoul: Ireseowon.

Moon, Hwarang, Jeonggyu Lee, Hyungik Kim, Seungeon Yang, Chunsung Lee, and Changhee Seo. 2020. *Regenerating Church: Till We Meet Again*. Seoul: Lifebook.

Nouwen, Henri J. M. 1997. *Adam: God's Beloved*. New York: Orbis Books.

Pivarnik, Gabriel. 2012. *Toward a Trinitarian Theology of Liturgical Participation*. Collegeville: Liturgical Press.

Polanyi, Micahel, and Harry Prosch. 1975. *Meaning*. Chicago: University of Chicago Press.

Polanyi, Michael. 1967. *The Tacit Dimension*. Garden City: Anchor.

Stieg, Cory. 2021. Bill Gates: 3 Innovations That Will Help America Get Ahead of the Next Pandemic. Available online: https://www.cnbc.com/2021/01/27/bill-gates-strategies-that-will-help-with-the-next-pandemic.html (accessed on 26 February 2021).

Swinton, John, and Harriet Mowat. 2006. *Practical Theology and Qualitative Research*. London: SCM.

Swinton, John. 2000. *Resurrecting the Person: Friendship and the Care of People with Mental Health Problems*. Nashville: Aingdon.

Thompson, Deanna A. 2020. Christ is Really Present, Even in Holy Communion via Online Worship. *Liturgy* 35: 18–24. [CrossRef]

Tylenda, Barbara, Jacqueline Beckett, and Rowland P. Barrett. 2007. Assessing Mental Retardation Using Standardized Intelligence Tests. *International Review of Research in Mental Retardation* 34: 27–97.

Volf, Miroslav. 1998. *After Our Likeness: The Church as the Image of the Trinity*. Grand Rapids: Eerdmans.

Vygotsky, Lev Semenovich. 1978. *Mind in Society: The Development of Higher Psychological Process*. Cambridge: Harvard University Press.

Wadell, Paul. 1994. Pondersing the Anomaly og God's love. In *Developmental Disabilities and Sacramental Access*. Edited by Edward Foley. Collegeville: Liturgical Press, pp. 53–72.

Webb-Mitchell, Brett. 2008. *Dancing with Disabilities: Opening the Church to All God's Children*. Eugene: Wipf &Stock.

Yong, Amos. 2007. *Theology and Down Syndrome: Reimagining Disability in Late Modernity*. Waco: Baylor University Press.

Zizioulas, John D. 2004. *Being as Communion*. New York: St. Vladimir's Seminary Press.

religions

MDPI

Article

Liturgical Participation: An Effective Hermeneutic for Individuals with Profound Memory Loss

Jared D. Yogerst

Independent Researcher and Chaplain, 620 California Ave. E., St. Paul, MN 55130, USA; jyogerst001@luthersem.edu

Abstract: In non-pandemic times adults with profound memory loss (PML) are isolated by virtue of the effects of their decline. The marginalization of this cohort has been greatly exacerbated by the present pandemic. Individuals and their caretakers are not seen as active members, but as objects of pastoral care. Leaving individuals outside of the present moment, PML makes it difficult to communicate or function. They may behave in ways that would be antithetical to their thinking. Individuals were isolated from their homes and worshiping communities. In this paper I will present a liturgical hermeneutic of Liturgical Participation. I will illustrate its effectiveness as a catechetical methodology for individuals experiencing PML. The methodology of Liturgical Participation will aid ministers in the work of raising the consciousness of individuals as active participants in the work of God.

Keywords: liturgy; liturgical studies; liturgical hermeneutics; reception; reception theory; sacramental theology; liturgical participation; Luther; Jauss

1. Introduction

The nursing home facility in which I work houses around 170 residents. Of those, many are experiencing varying levels of memory loss due to the myriad conditions that result in the symptoms of dementia. Many of these residents live in the several units in the building. For a select population experiencing profound memory loss (PML), there is the specialized memory care unit. This is a dedicated, and locked, unit for those individuals who require greater levels of specialized care. Individuals facing PML have experienced degrees of marginalization, stigmatization, and sidelining within society. Unfortunately, this has been the case even within communities of faith. Even within congregate care communities, PML populations can experience marginalization as communities of caregivers work to cope with behaviors while providing care to a fluid dynamic of residents and their individual expressions of PML.

Congregations, their pastors, and lay leaders may find PML members to be difficult to include within community activities. It can even be easier to simply sideline PML members, and their caregivers as, primarily, objects of care. This objectification further marginalizes PML members as non-participating in the liturgical life of the community. PML members may be unpredictable in their behaviors, even acting contrary to the community's norms. PML dislocates the individual from their current environment. It might make it difficult for PML members to engage with others or a liturgical activity to the degree they once did. Like their congregational counterparts, spiritual care workers in congregant care settings can participate in these same marginalizing activities. Congregational leaders and chaplains implicitly marginalize these groups by assessing PML members as incapable or disinterested in certain activities. An alternative marginalization is the objectification of PML members as primarily objects of care rather than fully participating liturgically and adding to, and thickening, the richness of the community's liturgical life. I would suggest that this marginalization is due to the concomitant effect of an implicit bias of ableism and a liturgical hermeneutic of reception based upon intellectual assent. This marginalization has been exacerbated by the present COVID-19 pandemic and its requisite lockdowns and social distancing obligations. These requirements in the time of COVID-19 exert pressures on both congregations and spiritual care within congregant care communities. I would suggest that an alternative hermeneutic that can provide verbiage to both spiritual leaders and lay people that moves beyond intellectual assent may mitigate the biases of ableism and cognitively contingent liturgical hermeneutics.

The hermeneutic I would like to suggest, Liturgical Participation, is based upon the dialogue of Reception Theory and Martin Luther's sacramental theology, called Sacramental Union. Liturgical Participation eschews the intellectual focus of the above bias in favor of the internal lifeworld of the liturgical participant engaged in dialogue with the lifeworld of the liturgical text. The *leitourgia* of worship is the work of God on behalf of the people, and therefore it is God's lifeworld made available and curated, with which the worshiper engages. Liturgical Participation as a liturgical hermeneutic strengthens the participatory benefits to both worshiper and presider. This hermeneutic benefits leaders to see PML members as fully participating and engaging with worship. Liturgical Participation is encouraging PML members themselves and their family members into receptivity of their fully participatory experience of God's promises made available in the Means of Grace. These individuals are fully engaged in worship as they progress through the stages of PML and are therefore valuable members of the community. They thicken the complexity and richness of their home communities and worshiping communities within congregate care centers. In this paper, I will provide a brief outline of the challenges facing PML members as they participate in worship. I will then, briefly, outline the dialogue partners of Jauss and Luther. I will then close with a brief outline of possible applications of Liturgical Participation and discuss the effectiveness of this hermeneutic for challenging the marginalization of PML members in their communities of worship.

2. Profound Memory Loss

PML is a complex and varied disease. While Alzheimer's is the most common form, dementia comes in many forms. Even within those forms, how it effects the individual is varied and over time can progress at different rates. However, the end stage of the disease is always the same. PML is always terminal. According to the Alzheimer's Association there are three stages to PML that progressively degrade both memory and physical capacity as the brain's capability to access neuropathways diminishes.[1] The first (mild) stage may not be noticeable to others, but is associated with misplacing common objects or forgetting words. An individual in the mild stage may be able to continue to work and drive; they are still capable of being independent. The second (moderate) stage is marked by an increasing dependence on the care of others. This second stage tends to be the longest and can span years. The final (severe) stage creates the greatest level of dependence and will require ever-present care. At this stage the communicative level has become heavily impaired. The individual may not be aware of their surroundings, and is no longer oriented to person, place, and time. These pervasive effects of PML are caused by their isolation, both from others and from themselves. The COVID-19 pandemic has provided an opportunity for further isolation of this population, even within congregant care facilities.

The present social constraints of the COVID-19 pandemic have combined with the socially isolating nature of PML to further marginalize this community. As communities of all types contend with social distancing obligations, PML individuals have become further isolated. Communities of faith moved their faith practices to online platforms. These online platforms are difficult for older adults to navigate. Imagine the impossibility of PML individuals attempting to access online services. Even within congregant care

[1] (The Alzheimer's Association 2020a).

facilities, social distancing obligations have greatly curtailed group settings. Residents are not able to visit with family and friends within the facility nor visit outdoor spaces or their former homes on leave of absence. Pastors and other congregational leaders are no longer able to visit residents within these facilities. Even within congregant care facilities, communal dining is no longer the norm. Nursing and support staff are stretched thin with needing to provide closer individualized support to socially distanced residents. Added to the increased workload is the increased anxiety for staff about contracting the illness, especially by those considered high risk. The pandemic exacerbates the ways in which PML individuals are isolated and marginalized even within systems that are intended to aid and support them. Spiritual care leaders must be more aware of this isolation as the prevalence of dementia, especially Alzheimer's, is expected to grow in the coming decades.

Anticipated increases in Alzheimer's and other kinds of dementia diagnosis means PML is a growing concern to communities of faith. According to the Alzheimer's Association, 5.8 million people 65 years and older are experiencing Alzheimer's dementia.[2] In just five years there will be a projected 22% increase in Alzheimer's diagnosis in the United States.[3] By 2050 the total number of Alzheimer's diagnoses will be 13.8 million.[4] With these projected increases, it is imperative that leaders in faith communities orient towards inclusive views of participation in worship in order to mitigate the isolating effects of ableist biases. Attending to these individuals, as well as their caregivers and family members, in such a way as they are not simply objects of pastoral care will enrich both the community as well as the lives of PML sufferers and their loved ones. It is necessary to be aware of and cope with the consequent challenges posed by PML to best curate the liturgical activity for the differently abled.

The dual biases of ableism and a hermeneutic based upon intellectual assent can hinder how members with PML are viewed as fully participating in the community's acts of worship. Ryan et al. illustrate the issues facing PML individuals within communities of faith, "While individuals with dementia clearly have increased physical needs over a normally aging adult, the mere presence of these needs negatively alters the way they are perceived and treated by others ... "[5] Problematizing PML sufferers marginalizes them as objects of care, otherizing them as opposed to the *undamaged* us. This marginalization diminishes both the individuals with PML and their communities of faith. It is, therefore, fortuitous that observational studies illustrate that individuals experiencing PML function the highest in environments in which they are personalized.[6] According to a meta-analysis of studies on lived space, the concepts of belonging, meaningfulness, safety and security, and autonomy were important to individuals with PML and encouraged personalization. [7] The authors noted, "The comprehensive understanding of the categories described is captured by the latent theme: 'Living with dementia is similar to living in a space where the walls keep closing in.'"[8] Dementia narrows the lives of those enduring the progress of the disease. The above categories provide ways in which to expand the individual's lived environment and developing this hermeneutic can be a point of contact in that regard. If Liturgical Participation is to be a useful hermeneutic to PML individuals, these above criteria ought to be presentable in the dialogue of the interior world of the worshiper and God. Liturgical Participation may aid in supporting the lucidity of individuals experiencing PML and supporting their comfort by advancing belonging, meaningfulness, safety and security, and autonomy by attuning faith leaders to the experience of a narrowed world.

2 (The Alzheimer's Association 2020b, p. 18).
3 (Ibid., p. 24).
4 (Ibid., p. 14).
5 (Ryan et al. 2005, p. 46).
6 (Holton 2016, p. 259).
7 (Hege Forsund et al. 2018).
8 (Ibid., p. 27).

3. Liturgical Participation

The hermeneutic of Liturgical Participation utilizes the works of Hans Robert Jauss in his Reception Theory as well as the Sacramental Union of Martin Luther. Liturgical Participation provides an opportunity to eschew the intellectually focused hermeneutic of participation used by many westerners. Andrew Sloan's narratively based theory of personhood situates this conversation within an ontologically appropriate view. Sloan's ontology situates identity within the participation of the individual within their own story, the stories of home communities, and the story of God. This relational-participatory view of personhood provides us with a departure point for the necessity of Liturgical Participation as a hermeneutic for liturgy, especially for those with PML and their circles of influence. Sloan's ontology closely parallels the categories of Forsund et al. and the necessity of repersonalizing the world of individuals experiencing PML. The strength of Liturgical Participation is the repersonalizing effect of the meeting of God's horizon with our own internal horizon in the liturgical event.

Sloan's suggestion of a narratively relational personhood presupposes an embodied quality of our humanness, and therefore our value to God and others. This view of personhood eschews the intellectual focus of our current social bias. Sloan writes, " … We are embodied beings, and it is as bodies that we experience the world and enter into relationships."[9] It is our embodiment, our interconnectedness and interdependence to others and to God, that curates our being, and therefore it is not something that can be lost, even with the insidious declines of dementia.

Luther and Jauss act as dialogue partners in the development of the hermeneutic of Liturgical Participation. Liturgical Participation captures the Aesthetic Experience of a worshiper engaged in dialogue with the life of God.[10] Jauss uses the term *lifeworld* to describe the essential phenomenological core of both the reader and the text. The lifeworld, or horizon, of the text in the case of the liturgical text is God's life. God's horizon is made inhabitable by the appropriateness of the liturgical text. The worshiper engages with this inhabitable world. God's lifeworld is God's own horizon or world view. [11] The worshiper has found his or her own lifeworld to be inadequate to understand his or her experience in the world.[12] In a given text, if appropriate, the worshiper finds ways of understanding these life experiences that cohere better to the world than his or her current internal horizon.

Jauss follows the writing of Hans Georg Gadamer in his understanding of the present activity of the curation of the interior world of the text. For both Gadamer and Jauss, this interior world made available is not a recapitulation of a past event, nor an entirely new world.[13] Instead, the interior world of the text is curated by the dialogue between reader and text and is made new again within each interaction. This dialogue is called the Aesthetic Experience. The Aesthetic Experience is like the meeting of old friends in a new interplay in the sharing of stories and emotions. The reader attunes to the lifeworld of the text because an appropriate text answers the questions posed by the reader in a dialogue. Relating to the text dialogically aids in the curation of a new internal horizon that better responds to the reader's experience. Jauss writes:

In a manner of speaking, Aesthetic Experience is effective both in utopian foreshadowing and in retrospective recognition. It perfects the imperfect world not merely by projecting future experience but also by preserving past experience which could continue

9 (Sloan 2019, p. 146).
10 (Yogerst 2019).
11 Throughout this paper I utilize several terms interchangeably. The reader may find it helpful for me to explain the terms further. The terms: internal horizon, lifeworld, and world view, all adhere to a concept common in the hermeneutics of Reception Theory and its cousin, Reader Response Theory. These three terms are used to capture the conception that the perspectives of reader and author are caught up in their personal point of view, personal experiences, historical view, and communities of influence. The task of interpretation is the cohesion or conflict between the varying horizons that connect between reader and author. The strength of Jauss' Reception Theory is his insistence that these horizons should not be overcome. The interaction of the various horizons should be leveraged by the reader to better interpret the text.
12 (Yogerst 2019, p. 365).
13 (Thiselton 1980, p. 299).

unrecovered along the path of mankind, were it not for the luminosity of a poetry and art which transfigures and monumentalizes it.[14]

The Aesthetic Experience is curative to the misapplication of the internal horizons of the reader. The reader's understanding of the world is incomplete or misapplied, and therefore, in their dialogue with the text, the reader hopes to come away with a new horizon that can be more effective in its application in the world. In the case of the liturgical text, the inhabitable world presented is God's life made possible by God's arrival in God's promises.

For a liturgical text, the horizon being met is God's horizon because what we call the liturgy is the administration of God's Means of Grace. The incipient presence of God's lifeworld differs from encounter or anamnesis as it is neither that Christ is simply present, nor is it simply remembering the event of the cross. The Aesthetic Experience is making available Christ's promises and their application in, with, and under the existential anxiety of the worshiper engaged in dialogue with the God revealed in the backwards nature of the bloody cross. Jauss's reception theory parallels well with Luther's sacramentality in that God's self-revelation is only found in the Means of Grace. It is the access to the promises of Christ that makes the Aesthetic Experience of Liturgical Participation existentiality curative. The arrival of God's promises in, with, and under the Means of Grace is the inhabitable world of God on behalf of the worshiper.

In Luther's work, the Aesthetic Experience is equivalent to the Happy Exchange. In the Happy Exchange the believer is united to Christ by faith. This uniting is motivated by the existential dread of a life separated from God fleshed out in the mind of the Christian by the accusations of the Law. In faith, the believer's fallen nature is exchanged for Christ's righteousness and Christ's multiple benefits.[15] Luther compares the uniting of the believer to Christ to that of Christ's promises united to the physical substance of the. Luther writes on the sacrament of the altar, "Here, too, out of two kinds of objects a union has taken place, which I shall call a 'Sacramental Union,' because Christ's body and the bread are given to us as a sacrament."[16] Luther's Happy Exchange parallels Jauss' Aesthetic Experience. The reader/worshiper perceives her worldview as inadequate to understand the world around her. In her existential crises, the worshiper turns to the lifeworld of God curated in the promises of Christ, available in the liturgy. Because the Aesthetic Experience is predicated by the inadequacies of the internal horizon of the worshiper, which motivates the engagement with God's lifeworld, the worshiper exits the Aesthetic Experience with a transformed internal horizon. They have integrated this engagement with God into their internal horizon to better interact with the world around them.

The Aesthetic Experience of Liturgical Participation is eminently repeatable. Its specificity and personal peculiarity eschew the intellectual focus of the ableism described earlier. Consequently, utilizing this hermeneutic would provide a departure point of full participatory potential irrespective of the perceived capabilities of the participants. This frees both presider and worshipers to let God show up how God wills. In this case, irrespective of capacity, the worshiper inhabits God's life, not based upon their own capacities, but because God approaches the worshiper. It is God who performs the *leitourgia*. The inhabitability of the Aesthetic Experience is motivated by God's arrival on behalf of humanity. For individuals facing PML, this allows them to show up how they will. Its repeatability means the Aesthetic Experience can be engaged over the lifetime—ever changing and ever repeating. Liturgical Participation is an appropriate way to address both the narrowing horizons of individuals with PML as well as the biases of faith leaders and laity.

14 (Jauss 1982, p. 10).

15 (Ibid., p. 365).

16 *Confession Concerning Christ's Supper* (1528), in Luther (1955, vol. 37, p. 300).

4. Practical Examples

Utilizing the approach of Liturgical Participation necessitates both active curation of the liturgical event and the work of consciousness raising in both the presider as well as the worshiping community. Consciousness raising is the attempt to bring people to awareness of an issue or concept. The presider's practice with individuals experiencing PML may move across both traditional parish settings as well as congregate care settings. This will provide a beginning conversation to see how a pastor can utilize Liturgical Participation in a mystagogical and practical way. I would like to provide examples of the task of consciousness raising, and an example of three liturgical events I have used in my own congregant care setting.

Consciousness raising for both a ministry leader, as well as the congregation, encourages awareness and attunement to what God is up to within the liturgical event. The goal of consciousness raising is not to make the liturgical event more holy or more effective. Raising the awareness of both presider and the worshiping community to what God is up to allows for the opportunity of connection. The community gathered in worship is presented with the arrival of Christ and his promises. Attunement to that event encourages the widening of the view of the worshipers. It encourages elasticity and resilience in thinking and feeling and the connecting of the worshiper's dialogue with God to their own experience in the world. Attunement and elasticity are engaged and encouraged when presiders purposefully utilize the historical and scriptural nuance of Christian worship. For many worshipers, there is a disconnect between Christian worship and *real life*. When the minister is attuned to the realness of worship, the minister is situated, historically and theologically, to guide the attunement of the worshiping community.

Across the many denominations of Christianity there is greater and lesser familiarity with the historic and scriptural roots of the myriad worship styles across those denominations. On their surface, some of those worship styles seem far removed from a historic liturgical style. Pastors and ministers across the spectrum of worshiping styles would benefit their communities by understanding the historical and scriptural sources and inspirations for their local style and habits. The work of attunement and consciousness raising is not the resurrection of a deceased golden age of liturgical life. Liturgical Participation begins with the rapprochement of pastors to their own history and sources from which they can then raise the consciousness and attunement of their community.

Presiders can commit to this mystagogical task by directly connecting hymn and song selection to scripture texts and sermon themes. Working to connect the efforts of small groups, Bible studies, Sunday school curriculum, and youth and family programs will provide a hedgerow around the common theme of God's promises made available in worship. The presider can also connect the Means of Grace, actively, within his or her sermon/homily. Raising consciousness among parish members might be connecting the entirety of the worship experience within the sending/benediction at the end of the service. Connecting the liturgical event as the compulsion to serve and act in the world attunes the worshiper to how Liturgical Participation is the impulse to be masks of God in the various vocations they inhabit during the week.

In my own setting, I have begun experimenting with ways in which to curate liturgical events through the Liturgical Participation lens. With PML residents particularly, I want to engage the categories identified by Forsund et al. of belonging, meaningfulness, safety and security, and autonomy. Curating liturgical events with these categories in mind may encourage lucidity and personalization of individuals with PML. There are three such groups that illustrate this in action. The three groups are: Hymn-Story, Bible Art, and Sights and Sounds of Faith.[17] These three groups provide a testing ground for

[17] In addition to daily group programming, I also produce a daily 20–30 min. video devotion that follows a similar pattern. These videos are broadcast within the building over the cable service.

Liturgical Participation as it relates to the categories Forsund et al. identify as important to repersonalization in the PML context.

My goal with these groups is to encourage remembering of older, formative, memories. Within the PML community, these older memories are more resilient. Each group emphasizes different senses and historic styles of worship. Within a congregant care community there is not always a clear hegemony of backgrounds and experience. Consequently, the presider may want to widen the historic sources used in curating liturgical events. Each group is approximately 30 min. On average a group has about 12–20 residents present. The meeting space is the common room in the memory care unit. Background noise and interruptions are frequent by staff and other residents coming in and out of the space. The theme is selected to connect to the Gospel lesson assigned for that week in the Revised Common Lectionary. Each week a single hymn and image is used for each video and in-person group.

The Hymn-Story group utilizes a single hymn to explore over the course of a single meeting. The same hymn is used throughout the broadcasted videos during the week as well. The group opens with an invocation, prayer, and reading of the Gospel lesson. During the program, I play two renditions of the song, preferably by different performers. Between playing the two renditions, I provide a short history or story about the hymn or hymn writer. After the second rendition, I do a short devotion connecting the Gospel reading to the hymn and the larger theme for the week. I break up this discussion looking for recognition or reactions from the residents and attempt to elicit expressions of feelings or memories associated with the hymn. The second program, Bible Art, approaches the same thing but with visual art rather than music.

Like the previous program, Bible Art is a 30-min. program based upon the Gospel lesson for the week and its corresponding theme. I choose a piece of historical art and utilize that as the center of the program. Bible Art starts with the same opening pattern as outlined above. In this case, the program is meant to stimulate visually based memories and emotions rather than auditory. In this program, I provide less historical background on the artwork and focus more on composition and style to evoke an emotion and connection to the theme. The third program attempts to utilize this hermeneutic in terms of the resident's experiences within their communities.

Sights and Sounds of faith combine both the auditory and visual stimulus of the previous two groups and focuses on the experiences of residents in unstructured church programming such as potlucks or youth events. The program is structured the same as above. In the body of the program the focus turns to sights and sounds of activities common in communal church activities. I have found autonomous sensory meridian response (ASMR) videos to be a close approximation of these experiences. ASMR is a genre of video that emphasizes sounds that have a high-tactile component to elicit a synesthesia response.[18] These videos have been used for relaxation, especially amid sensory overload. The ASMR video has the capability of situating the worshiper back in their embodied experiences. An example video I used was a family frying fish in oil. This video was associated with Ash Wednesday and the start of the Lenten fast.

Each of these programs is informed by the hermeneutic of Liturgical Participation and the goal of repersonalization as mentioned earlier. Utilizing this hermeneutic, parish leaders, members, individuals experiencing PML, and their loved ones can better curate liturgical events to encourage and redeem the full participation of the differently abled. Consciousness raising and specific curation of events will thicken and enrich the experience of the whole community.

[18] Synesthesia is the brain's connection of two different kinds of stimulation, so that the experience of one stimulus simultaneously triggers the neuropathways associated with the other stimulus.

5. Effectiveness of Liturgical Participation

The experience of PML is both the dysregulation of the self as well as the narrowing of the world of individual with PML. It is the case, then, that two roles for the Aesthetic Experience exists. The Aesthetic Experience curates an inhabitable world responsive to the questions of the worshiper. This inhabitable world provides for an externalized tool for self-regulation and the widening of the individual's world. Looking again at the themes outlined by Forsund et al. we can elucidate some possible questions being asked of God's life by the worshiper experiencing PML. Forsund et al. articulate the following important categories when considering the self-regulation of individuals experiencing PML: belonging, meaningfulness, safety and security, and autonomy. These categories allow for individuals experiencing PML to maintain their sense of self through their environment and maintain their self-regulation.

The curated life of God in liturgy is an opportunity to address Forsund's categories in the sacred space. Simplified and historically grounded aspects of liturgy, as well as narrowed choices, may seem counterintuitive if we imagine the PML individual as struggling with a narrowed world. PML is partly isolating because of the dislocation of the individuals from their present moment and time. In God's life it is a function of God's accessibility to the individual, not their capacity to intellectually assent or be emotionally present. Liturgical Participation is ideally situated to provide an external source for self-regulation and an expansiveness of time and place. The comfort provided by the curation of God's lifeworld is peculiar to this liturgical experience and is certainly repeatable. This hermeneutic redeems the isolating aspects of PML and leverages them to effect transformation for both the individual experiencing PML as well as her community around her. This redemption thickens the experiences of the community, eschews the ableism of our culture's worldview, and transforms horizons as Liturgical Participation better answers the questions posed by the multiplicity of worshipers.

The COVID-19 pandemic has created many new and unexpected barriers and opportunities to communities of faith. For those suffering with PML, there has been a greater exacerbation of isolation, loneliness, and a declining access to the very relationships and environments that encourage greater lucidity. We can utilize the concepts of belonging, meaningfulness, safety and security, and autonomy as a key to gauge how effective Liturgical Participation is as an hermeneutic within the context of PML. In the Aesthetic Experience these concepts are points of dialogue between the internal world of the worshiper and the world of the text. The inhabitable engagement with God is a lived space in which these questions can be posed. Exiting the Aesthetic Experience the worshiper is transformed as she or he integrates the answers received.

6. Conclusions

There is an issue of marginalization of individuals experiencing PML due to the perceived deficiencies of individuals with PML as well as the systematic challenges present within systems of care. These challenges have been exacerbated by the present social struggles in our world, as well as the COVID-19 pandemic. The hermeneutic of Liturgical Participation outlined here can provide a perspective on participation that highlights the activity of God engaging the individual as she is, in her present moment. It is this particularity that illustrates the helpfulness of this view in the present context. With this hermeneutic in mind the worshiper, presider, and communities of faith can see individuals experiencing PML as engaged in the life of God made available in liturgy. With this perspective, each worshiper is engaged for her own internal lifeworld rather than meeting an external threshold of capacity. Liturgical Participation is a helpful hermeneutic to understand how differently abled people can engage in worship, even as their capacities are uncommon within the community.

Funding: This research receive not external funding.

Data Availability Statement: No new data were created or analazed in this study. Data sharing is not applicable to this article.

Conflicts of Interest: The author declares no conflict of interest.

References

Hege Forsund, Linn, Ellen Karine Grov, Anne-Sofie Helvik, Lene Kristine Juvet, Kristi Skovdahl, and Siren Eriksen. 2018. The Experience of Living Space in Persons with Dementia: A Systematic Meta-Synthesis. *BMC Geriatrics* 18: 1–27. [CrossRef]

Holton, Richard. 2016. Memory, Persons and Dementia. *Studies in Christian Ethics* 29: 256–60. [CrossRef]

Jauss, Hans Robert. 1982. *Aesthetic Experience and Literary Hermeneutics*. Translated by Michael Shaw. Minneapolis: University of Minnesota Press.

Luther, Martin. 1955. *Luther's Works*. Edited by Jaroslav Pelikan, Helmut T. Lehmann and Christopher Boyd Brown. Philadelphia: Fortress Press, St. Louis: Concordia Publishing House, 75 vols.

Ryan, Ellen B., Lori Schindel Martin, and Amanda Beaman. 2005. Communication Strategies to Promote Spiritual Well-being among People with Dementia. *The Journal of Pastoral Care & Counseling* 59: 43–55.

Sloan, Andrew. 2019. The Dissolving Self? Dementia and Identity if Philosophical Theology. *Science and Christian Belief* 31: 131–50.

The Alzheimer's Association. 2020a. Available online: https://www.alz.org/alzheimers-dementia/stages (accessed on 1 January 2021).

The Alzheimer's Association. 2020b. Alzheimer's Facts and Figures 2020. *Journal of the Alzheimer's Association* 16: 391–460. [CrossRef] [PubMed]

Thiselton, Anthony C. 1980. *The Two Horizons: New Testament Hermeneutics and Philosophical Description with Special Reference to Heidegger, Bultmann, Gadamer, and Wittgenstein*. Grand Rapids: William B. Eerdmans Publishing Co.

Yogerst, Jar. 2019. The Re-Wilding of Worship: A Post-Contemporary Reception. *Word and World* 39: 362–70.

religions

MDPI

Article

Essential Workers, Essential Services? *Leitourgia* in Light of Lockdown

Bryan Cones

Pilgrim Theological College, University of Divinity, Parkville, VIC 3052, Australia; bmcones@gmail.com

Abstract: Within days of the outbreak of COVID-19, the language of "essential work" and "essential workers" became commonplace in public discourse. "Church workers" and their in-person liturgical services were largely deemed "non-essential", and most assemblies shifted worship to online platforms. While some reflection on this virtual "church work" has appeared in the intervening months, there has been less evaluation of the gathered assembly's absence from the public square, along with the contribution its liturgical work might offer in interpreting the pandemic and its effects. This essay imagines a post-COVID-19 agenda for liturgical studies that focuses on a recovery of Christian liturgy as public, in-person, and "essential" service done for the sake of the *polis*—a public example of "church doing world"—that proposes a countersign to the inequalities of contemporary consumer culture laid bare in these last months. It begins by engaging in dialogue with the *leitourgia* of groups who insisted on the essential nature of their public service, in particular the public protests against police violence that marked the summer of 2020. In doing so, it seeks ways liturgical assemblies might better propose a "public theology" of God's work in the world understood as the *concursus Dei*, the divine accompanying of creation and humanity within it.

Keywords: public theology; liturgy; eucharist; COVID-19; pandemic; assembly; liturgical theology; protest; Black Lives Matter

1. Introduction: What Is "Essential Work", and Who Bears Its Risks?

The outbreak of COVID-19 made immediately commonplace the language of what is "essential" in terms of both work and access to goods and services. Those judged "essential workers"[1] included health care providers, first responders, public servants, and many retail sector employees. This designation unveiled the relative value assigned to the work and workers required to maintain "the essential": Many roles are poorly compensated, and many workers belong to gender, racial, and ethnic groups that have suffered historic and systemic policies of inequality and exclusion. These "essential workers" were assigned to take the risk of providing essential services during the pandemic while simultaneously continuing to bear longstanding injustices based on race, gender, and class.[2]

"Church work" in its customary, in-person forms fell among what was deemed "non-essential" and thus exempt from such risks; churches were even forbidden from engaging them. My own context in this case was as pastor of a mid-size, suburban Episcopal church, which was primarily White, largely professional, financially secure with some exceptions, generally "progressive" in terms of politics and theological outlook, if not particularly

1 See, for example, the National Conference of State Legislatures' (2020) description of the broad range of work deemed "essential" across industries.

2 A U.S. National Institutes of Health Study, for example, connected the higher rates of death due to COVID-19 for non-Hispanic Blacks directly to their overrepresentation in occupations judged "essential", especially in the U.S. Midwest. Researchers conclude, "The racial disparities among essential workers in the United States that we highlight are a byproduct of longstanding systemic racism and structural inequalities, combined with a lack of public policy aimed at protecting the lives of essential workers who risk their lives daily to protect and/or provide for others" (Rogers et al. 2020, p. 321). The Institute for Policy Studies (2020a), a progressive think tank, provides a broad picture of the uneven effects of the pandemic across a range of marginalized populations.

politically active. Few of us were counted among the "essential workers", though virtually all members routinely interacted with such workers through their everyday economic activity.

Soon after the suspension of in-person worship, the congregation began a weekly Zoom "liturgy of the word",[3] which provided the primary moment of interpretation, first, of the pandemic with its uneven effects, and second, of the concurrent public responses to police violence against Black bodies. While some of our prayer did attempt to address those events, primarily through the preaching and intercessory "prayers of the people", its primary audience was members of the church. As I surveyed other local churches, especially others in my Episcopal diocese,[4] the judgment seemed to hold: From diocesan communications through to the congregational level, the prayer we engaged served primarily as pastoral care for those who took it up, both as a means of maintaining relational connections and of interpreting world events. While preaching and prayer inevitably addressed what was happening "out there", the conversation was limited to church members in relation to each other and God. It may have been "essential" to us, but likely to few others, nor did it directly engage the "essential workers" at the front lines of exposure to the pandemic and its effects.

What follows is my own attempt to interrogate the limited reach of much Christian liturgy during the COVID-19 pandemic beyond an assembly's members. It imagines a post-COVID-19 agenda for pastoral liturgical studies[5] that focuses on a recovery of Christian liturgy as public, in-person, and "essential" service done for the sake of the *polis*. In doing so, the assembly proposes a public example of "church doing world"[6] that actively engages the inequalities of consumer culture laid bare in these last months and proposes a countersign to the political and economic status quo. I take for granted that Christian liturgy is a form of "public theology"[7] in dialogue with the world around it undertaken by a "corporate theologian", the Christian assembly gathered as a "primary symbol"[8] that refracts God's work to the wider *polis*. It begins by engaging in dialogue with the *leitourgia* of the secular public protests that marked the summer of 2020 for ways liturgical assemblies might better propose their "public theology". It concludes by imagining a possible expression of such "essential" *leitourgia* from my then-context in an Episcopal Church in suburban Chicago, Illinois, U.S.

2. What "Work" Have We Been Doing, and for Whom?

Beyond my own context, broader reflection on liturgical prayer in an online environment echoes the contention that common prayer during the pandemic has been largely directed to church members. Among the topics producing widespread commentary, for example, is whether it is possible to celebrate "virtual eucharist", with concern primarily

3 My own reflections on our online attempts at common prayer can be found in "How Do We Gather Now? What We Have Lost—and Gained—through Virtual Worship" (Cones 2020a).

4 A representative example from my own local Episcopal bishop, Jeffrey Lee (2020), suffices, in which he encouraged the churches in his oversight to "a Lenten fast from public worship", which has since been renewed in various forms.

5 Domenico Sartore, developing the work of the late Mark Searle, describes "pastoral liturgical studies" as a three-step task: "(1) an empirical task: a phenomenological description of the event of celebration, explanation of the meaning of the words and deeds that constitute the rite, liturgical attitudes, and the specific assembly's receptiveness; (2) a hermeneutic task: how symbols work and how symbolic language communicates, and whether our contemporaries effectively engage in communication with them; (3) a critical task: comparison with the results of other disciplines, critical evaluation of the various forms of religious imagination in the various churches, and identification of the various forms in which contemporary liturgy can be alienated and alienating" (Sartore 1998, p. 71). See also Searle (1983).

6 The expression evokes Aidan Kavanagh's oft-quoted claim that liturgy "play[s] extremely hard ball with the world by remaining clearheaded about what the world can and cannot do for itself." Just prior Kavanagh notes, apropos of the current pandemic, "*Orthodoxia* has every reason to regard a child dead of war or starved by poverty as anything but normal" (Kavanagh 1984, pp. 158–59).

7 Elaine Graham provides a helpful guide to the genre of public theology, with a nod to the possibility that liturgy might find a place on her "map": "Public theology has a 'performative' dimension, since actions may speak louder than words" (Graham 2020, p. 14). Edward Foley (2008) gives a more fulsome articulation of the connection between liturgy and public theology. More recently, James Farwell (2020) describes liturgy as a "formation" for public theologians.

8 This expression reflects the contention of Robert Hovda through his many "Amen Corner" columns in the journal *Worship*. It was most clearly stated in a document of the U.S. Bishops' Committee on the Liturgy (1977, para. 28), Environment and Art in Catholic Worship: "Of all the symbols with which the liturgy deals, none is more important than this assembly of believers." See also Hovda (1988).

for church members deprived of communion. Most Anglican, Lutheran, and Reformed denominational level reflection has discouraged these practices,[9] drawing attention to the necessity of embodied gathering as the *sine qua non* of eucharist in particular (though not necessarily of other forms of liturgical prayer) and encouraging a focus on the presence of Christ in the proclaimed scripture. Other commentators have taken a different approach, with Deanna Thompson (2020) arguing that, although mediated by technology, a virtual gathering remains embodied. Diana Butler Bass has protested what she judges to be a "forced fast", contending that "the church"—by which she apparently means the clergy—"has been, in effect, hoarding the bread and wine, restraining the healing beauty of Eucharist when hungry people most need to feast" (Butler Bass 2020). While these arguments may make sense among some Christians, David Jacobsen argues that "to ecclesial outsiders", such debates may "tend to read like the premise of some home decorating shows on cable: what should be the center of the room, the framed Chagall print or the family heirloom reading desk on the opposite wall?" (Jacobsen 2018, pp. 372–73).

Taken as a whole, then, most liturgical prayer in response to COVID-19 and reflections upon it have focused on the effect of the suspension in gathering on Christian communities. There has been comparatively less reflection on the loss of the assembly's *leitourgia* in the public sphere, its "essential work" proposing the reign of God as an alternative to the current economic and political order. Nevertheless, the consumer economy has continued to function more or less without major interruption, its inequities further magnified by the pandemic. However, maintaining it has been judged worth the risk of infection among "essential workers". Their work has yielded immense profits for a few, exacerbating the already overwhelming wealth and income divide across the very race, class and gender lines traced in the judgment of what is "essential work".[10]

The narrow focus among many church commentators on the eucharistic elements or even their absence suggests "eucharist" as yet another "consumable" product functioning, in the words of Carvalhaes, "in tandem, with or against, the economic order" (Carvalhaes 2017, p. 471), though as Belcher (2020) notes, that connection is often veiled. In this case, eucharist does not particularly disrupt or interrogate the marketplace and its effects.[11] This congruity calls to mind Daniel Rhodes' (2020) commentary on the failure of Christian liturgy to engage "disaster capitalism", through which public goods are privatized to generate profit in response to disaster. Rhodes sees a need for "a liturgy interfused with a counter-politics" (Rhodes 2020, p. 95), but it would be hard to argue that many churches' "public service" has yet risen to this task in the matter of COVID, much less been ready to bear the risks that might be involved in doing so. This is arguably a "pre-existing condition," as Carvalhaes (2017, p. 466) makes clear in his description of a "dichotomy" in much liturgical and theological thinking between *doxa* and *praxis*, between congregational prayer and Christian engagement with the world.[12] This was likely no less true before the pandemic, but its widespread yet uneven effects and the inequalities it has magnified have laid bare the limited ability of most Christian *leitourgia* to propose a divine alternative to the economic status quo.

[9] These reflections are both widespread and widely available. By and large, denominational bodies and theologians have discouraged attempts to celebrate eucharist without gathering in person. See, for example, the Episcopal Church's Presiding Bishop Michael Curry' (2020) statement, "On Our Theology of Worship"; the Evangelical Lutheran Church in America' (2020) "Worship in Times of Public Health Concerns: COVID-19/Coronavirus"; and "Using Our Rites and Resources" (Anderson et al. 2020) offered by "theologians and scholars of Methodist worship." Gribben (2020) offers a helpful and wide-ranging evaluation of these in his comments on The Uniting Church in Australia's decision to permit celebration of online communion. See also The Uniting Church in Australia (2020), "Temporary Arrangements for Holy Communion".

[10] Institute for Policy Studies (2020b) summarizes the results of studies that document an increase of $1 trillion among U.S. billionaires through December 2020.

[11] Kimberly Hope Belcher argues that there is a direct, if often concealed, connection between sacramental and everyday economic exchanges, with the former proposing a eschatological subversion of the latter: "The Christian sacramental revelation is not the separation of the eschatological from the worldly, but the subversion of the worldly into the eschatological" (Belcher 2020, pp. 17–19).

[12] Elsewhere, Carvalhaes (2020) echoes Tissa Balasuriya, who more than 40 years ago asked, "Why is it that in spite of hundreds of thousands of eucharistic celebrations, Christians continue as selfish as before? Why have the 'Christian' Mass going peoples been the most cruel colonizers of human history?" (Balasuriya 1977, p. 2).

At first glance, such challenges seem beyond the reach of any assembly's *leitourgia*, no matter how well intentioned. Nonetheless, as many have argued, Christian liturgy has functioned throughout the ages—for better and for worse—as public acts of theological interpretation, which interact in the public square with those proposed by others.[13] Hilton Scott (2020b) argues that the pandemic has thrust assemblies into an unusual experience of liminality, in which their primary public theology is no longer able to function as it generally has. He sees this time, and I agree, as a creative, open space for assemblies to seek new forms of contextual *koinonia* and *communitas*, which, in light of the pandemic, received liturgical practices appear limited in their ability to propose.[14] A promising place to engage this creative space is in dialogue[15] with those who refused to comply with the public orders to suspend their *leitourgia* in response to the inequalities unveiled in this time. What adjustments do they propose to Christian liturgy that might amplify an assembly's "public service", even render it "essential"?

3. Learning from Others' *Leitourgia*

Among those refusing to comply with restrictions on in-person gatherings were the millions who gathered to protest police violence against Black bodies. My participation in one of these stirred my own thinking about the *leitourgia* of the churches, a strategy Sharon Fennema (2018) has deployed in her own reflections on marches protesting gentrification in Oakland, California.[16]

The march in question gathered several thousand people in Chicago's Lakeview neighborhood, a center of LGBTQIA+ culture and entertainment. It is, however (as organizers pointed out), one with a history of excluding Black and transgender members of the rainbow. Notably, a majority of those gathered were non-Black, which became clear as the protest unfolded and reflected the city's well-documented racial segregation by "neighborhood",[17] of which I am a part as a White resident of the city's majority White North Side.[18]

A number of elements would be familiar to anyone in a church on Sunday. First were the litanies that accompanied the mile-long procession, dominated by "Say their/her/his name", depending on the gender identity of the victim of police violence being named. These were interspersed with broadly familiar chants that mark civil rights protests ("no justice, no peace", "this is what democracy looks like"). The cumulative effect echoed liturgical lament,[19] though in this predominantly White North Side assembly, it also had the feel of a confession—perhaps in response to a "call" from the march's

13 As Edward Foley notes, "Whether we agree with it or not, societies, cultures, and even countries are already promulgating their own public theologies" (Foley 2008, p. 41).

14 Hilton Scott proposes in his South African context a renewed understanding of the concept of *ubuntu* ("I am because we are") in light of the indiscriminate nature of COVID-19 infection, "a new status quo that is fully human and therefore able to accept difference and otherness as well as navigate such relationships without discriminating" (Scott 2020b).

15 Foley argues that dialogue is key to public theology proposed through liturgy, "not simply supplying answers to questions and problems posed by the world, but ritually responsive in the ways it symbolizes, celebrates, and consecrates God's brooding Spirit afoot in the liturgy of the world" (Foley 2008, p. 47).

16 The connections between liturgy and public protest have long been a thread in liturgical theology, if underdeveloped, at least as a matter of most congregational practice. Harold Leatherland, for example, argues, "I am predisposed to the view that protest is not alien to liturgy, that protest can be uttered liturgically, and that liturgy itself can be considered, from some aspects, as protest" (Leatherland 1974, p. 18).

17 The reality and effects of racial segregation in Chicago's "city of neighborhoods" are well-documented. See, for example, the joint report of the Metropolitan Planning Council and Urban Institute (2017), "The Cost of Segregation: Lost Income. Lost Lives. Lost Potential."

18 Michael Jaycox (2017, pp. 307–9) notes the importance of acknowledging the social location one brings to a direct action, particularly as a White person and academic at a Black Lives Matter protest, including the dangers of appropriating the stories of those marginalized by race, gender, or class. For my own part, as a White, queer, and cisgender male Chicagoan, I joined this protest as a regular visitor and participant in the culture of Lakeview, and thus see myself as complicit in the injustices raised in the protest, which I also hope to resist and repair.

19 Burns (2020) explores the interaction of confession (directed toward individual actions) and lament ("confessing more than sin," or its larger manifestations) in Christian assemblies through the work of Gail Ramshaw. While the former is quite common across the traditions, Burns finds fewer of the latter (apart from Ramshaw's work), which limits many assemblies in their ability to name and mourn much of the inequality the pandemic has unveiled. See also Ramshaw (2017, pp. 22–27). Suna-Koro (2019, p. 34) proposes a recovery of lament as a "a profoundly counter-hegemonic liturgical practice that can empower Christians to name and subvert the polarizing imaginaries of dehumanization, resentment, and hostility" characteristic of anti-migrant and racist policies.

Black leadership.[20] The embodied juxtaposition between call and response refracted through those racialized identities calls to mind Carvalhaes's identification of the limits of most "generalized" denominational confessions, which "seldom make us think about real reparations to Black and Indigenous people" (Carvalhaes 2020, p. 30). Unlike most church litanies, however, these arose from various groups within the processing assembly and were often modified in the chanting and were not directed from "the front". Whatever the character of the litany, it arose from the "body", not from the "head". It evoked Aidan Kavanagh's description of the "many-to-many" interaction characteristic of liturgical prayer as a "social occasion" (the protest) (Kavanagh 1984, pp. 137–39), which he distinguishes from the "one-to-many" interaction of a lecture hall or the "one-to-one" character of a personal conversation. Kavanagh notes that one of the purposes of such a many-to-many "social occasion" is that it produces an "effective symbol of social survival" (Kavanagh 1984, p. 137). This description is particularly apropos of the protest as a "ritual or quasi-liturgical" activity that allows those gathered to "construct and become a narrative-based collective" (Jaycox 2017, p. 310).

Once the procession arrived at a major intersection, the organizer shifted to "presider", directing this assembly's attention, proposing and modeling what to do, and yielding to other voices. The call to order began with the presider inviting any Black persons present to come "up to the front", with the rest of the assembly parting to create an aisle and spontaneously applauding as Black and transgender persons filtered forward. Their appearance at the end of the procession suggested to me the customary place of the vested ordained ministers in an Episcopal procession. While I fear it appears clerical there, in this case, it seemed a felicitous "ordering" of the assembly, with Black and transgender bodies proposed as privileged norms within a primarily White and presumably cisgender assembly.

The presider then proposed the equivalent of an embodied ritual action, instructing those gathered to kneel on the pavement and hold a nearly nine-minute silence to recall George Floyd's suffocation. While I have experienced such silences in Christian liturgy, the "sacred space" created by contact with asphalt and the press of people gave it a profound anamnetic character, both "embodied and empathetic", that Fennema finds in Oakland. While it echoed one particular "crucifixion", it refracted those terrible minutes in a way that made present countless others; it further proposed a vicarious identification with its victims among those, such as myself, who had never experienced its direct effects. As Fennema writes, it was an act of "remembrance and imagination, when we begin to make the connection between the experience of others and our own in a way that affects us ... reclaiming the space and making visible the people—the many faces of Christ—who have been suppressed or erased" (Fennema 2018, p. 385). Though displaced from Minneapolis, the asphalt common to every American city combined with the bodies pressed against it evoked the character of a liturgical "real symbol",[21] The action effectively made present the place of Floyd's death and referred further to Chicago's own places of similar deaths.

4. Adjusting an Assembly's "Public Service"

This example of protest suggests to me some dimensions of liturgical practice that need attention if liturgies are to offer the "essential public service" of a countersign to the political and economic status quo. First among these is a shift in mentality for many assemblies, my own included: We must adopt the attitude that, like a public protest, our work is directed primarily to the *polis*, not the *ekklesia*. The purpose of being "called out" is to render a "public service" so essential that "salvation", incarnationally manifested in

20 While this interpretation is my own conjecture, one of Jaycox (2017, p. 320) interviewees, "Alice", who is Black, wondered if White protesters want Black participants "to absolve them of their sin".

21 Michael Skelley, interpreting Karl Rahner, describes a "real symbol" as the "the supreme and primal form of representation in which one reality renders another really present" (Skelley 1991, p. 38). Jaycox (2017, p. 312) also argues that protest is "symbolic action," which "has the power to mediate the world that can and should exist, but does not yet exist in its fullness, but which through ritual participation in the action already begins to break into our reality."

the flourishing of those made marginal, depends on it. This will likely require a shift in attitude from seeing worship as the assembly's work offered to God to understanding it as the *leitourgia* God's Spirit is groaning to do for the world through the assembly.

Building on that shift in attitude, the correlative need to adjust[22] the assembly's common action and the manner of its address in prayer becomes clear. I would argue that the relative passivity of many assemblies in relation to the world is directly related to the passivity they experience in most liturgical celebrations: Most remain "in their places" from beginning to end; any "marching" is limited to a few designated for that purpose and "chanting" is carefully ordered to certain voices. If liturgy is to be not only an act of public theology or, as Sally Brown (2013) describes it, formation in "discerning the public presence of God", the manner of its celebration is every bit as important as the words it voices.

Brown's concern about the weak connection between liturgical practices and public forms of action[23] suggests a need for more accessible "ritual vernacular" (to accompany linguistic ones).[24] Such common embodied action can propose the essential relationship between Christian liturgy and Christian mission as manifestations of the church's participation in the *missio Dei,* which Duraisingh describes as "the already up-and-running mission of God in the world" (Duraisingh 2010, p. 10). While that might lead to an assembly undertaking a public act akin to a protest,[25] an imagination shaped to make that connection needs a regular embodied *poiesis*—a ritual vernacular—to, in the words of Charles Fensham, "aid in the formation of collective identity, the creation of free space, the harnessing of emotions, and the shaping of a culture of advocacy and change" (Fensham 2016, p. 158).

In the matter of gathering, then, whenever possible, a more porous entrance from outside the church is in order. In the assembly I served, the "opening procession" obscured this connection by beginning and ending "indoors", from the front of the space for worship, to the back, and up front again. Nothing suggested the completion of a gathering bearing the "liturgy of the world"[26] "in" from "out there".

A fairly straightforward adjustment would be to begin outside and include a more representative procession not limited to those members of the assembly who have roles of leadership. To the extent that such a procession "orders" the assembly, it should reflect as much as possible the differences gathered, particularly those marginalized either outside or within it. Every assembly bears differences that are shunted to the side or excluded, whether based on age or ability or neurological function, not to mention race and cultural heritage. I have argued elsewhere (Cones 2020b) that these qualities are part of the "text" of any liturgy that can serve as sources for its public theology. The shape of an assembly's gathering is, in the words of Carvalhaes, an opportunity to "ascribe worthiness, or honor, to somebody or something" (Carvalhaes 2017, p. 477) as the street protest did in calling forward the Black and transgender members of that assembly. Despite the real risks of failure in the Christian assembly, for example, the danger of "tokenism", the gathering is a moment for an assembly to state what qualities in itself it proposes to value, particularly differences that have been made marginal.

22 I use this term deliberately to evoke Aidan Kavanagh's definition of liturgical theology: "the adjustment to deep change caused in the assembly by its being brought regularly to the brink of chaos in the presence of the living God." See Kavanagh (1984, p. 74).

23 Jaycox (2017, p. 339), more trenchantly than Brown, laments that "Catholic practices of incorporation have tended to, at best, capitulate to, or, at worst, amplify and affirm the habituating power of white supremacy," a judgment that could also be applied to my own Episcopal context.

24 Judith Kubicki, among others, argues that liturgical meaning is "primarily non-discursive and exhibitive. That is, meaning is not asserted by means of propositional content in worship, but exhibited or manifested in the interplay of symbolic activity" (Kubicki 2006, p. 15). Thus, while the pandemic, its effects, and responses to it may have appeared in "discursive" forms in many liturgies (in preaching and prayers), these meanings lacked an accessible, non-discursive analog in ritual. Fensham argues that ritual, in this case Christian liturgy, can do so by bringing "a kind of insight with wider and more encompassing ethical and moral implications" (Fensham 2016, p. 160).

25 There are many examples of "liturgies after the liturgy" documented by both scholars and practitioners, though I would suggest these remain exceptional among the majority of churches. See, for example, Stewart (2012); Nóda (2017); and Scott (2020a).

26 Karl Rahner proposes God's self-disclosure in creation as "the terrible and sublime liturgy, breathing of death and sacrifice, which God celebrates and causes to be celebrated in and through human history in its freedom," which Christian liturgy symbolizes, reflects upon, and interprets. See Rahner (1976, pp. 179–80). See also Skelley (1991, pp. 133–58).

As to the word and song that gather the assembly, while the "chants" may differ from those found at a protest, the manner of their leadership and performance could better correspond to it. The "call to order", for example, need not originate from the same voice; indeed, in the case of a procession with some already "in place" and some moving through, the dialogue might be between those groups, laying the groundwork for the "many-to-many" interactions of the liturgy as it unfolds. Intercessory prayer offers further opportunity for active, communal engagement beyond their content. The diversity of voices that entered the room needs refraction in its prayers for the world. There is no reason beyond the logistics of finding enough willing voices for there to be a single "prayer leader", nor to restrict the prayers themselves to what is printed on a page. The Korean prayer pattern Tongsung Kido,[27] which includes an invitation to prayer, space for intercession from the assembly's members, and a sung response has promising possibilities for contextualizing such "prayer of the people".

After such prayers, most assemblies of my experience turn to the table and its proposal of *communitas* or *koinonia* within and beyond the gathered group. This turn is harder to discern in the *leitourgia* of public protest, though Fennema (2018, pp. 383–84) proposes the concept of "pilgrimage" as one promising analog. Nevertheless, the nine minutes of silence held by with the "real symbol" of all those bodies pressed to pavement did evoke a unity-across-difference, though perhaps without proposing its reconciliation. Regardless of its intent, it embodied a compelling "ritual vernacular" available across differences of race, class, wealth, gender, orientation, age. It suggested a "real symbol" of what M. Shawn Copeland has called "a praxis of solidarity" (Copeland 2010, pp. 124–28), which she connects to eucharist, embodied at an intersection and in the intersections of those gathered. How often do Christian assemblies render their eucharistic "public service" in such accessible and compelling ways?

What may be lacking in many assemblies is the "ritual vernacular" that makes the connection between the eucharist and the hunger of the world[28] (or in one's own backyard) a more accessible dimension of the assembly's imagination. Put plainly, if the *poiesis* of eucharist had been doing its "essential public service" all along, there would be no hunger at all, at least within reach of any who celebrate it. Nevertheless, the (pre-existing) hunger starkly exposed in the pandemic also reveals the relatively weak effect much eucharistic *leitourgia* has had on the hunger it is meant to contest. Belcher (2020) suggests this limit in imagination is the result of a "concealment" of the connection between sacramental eucharistic practice and everyday economic activity, which I would argue has analogs in the practice of many assemblies: It is often difficult to identify the food placed on the altar with what is plucked from the grocery shelf, much less the divine and human exchanges Belcher identifies in both.

An embodied expression unveiling these relationships, like the march that gathered the assembly, surely must include more than a few representatives bearing meager "gifts" rendered invisible by their containers and handed over to the clergy at a distant table. An assembly might start by never again using something called "a host" in favor of actual food, that is, real bread and wine or other culturally appropriate analogs that meet actual hunger. A more fulsome procession of full hands bearing a wider range of gifts would better propose a "vernacular" real symbol of a meal able to feed everyone and an economy refracting divine abundance. This must surely include the assembly pressing close to its own table—the infrastructure of the meal analogous to the asphalt of the city liturgy—to experience its own eucharistic solidarity with all who hunger.

27 This practice is commended by Alexander (1992, p. 445). See also Cones (2018).

28 This expression evokes Monika Hellwig' (1992) classic study on eucharist and hunger (originally published in 1976). See also Bieler and Schottroff (2007).

A eucharistic practice with a more outward turn might also call into question any "fencing" of the meal: While "open table" practice[29]—in which any who wishes can receive communion—disrupts the expectation of baptism before communion, it also suggests a broader catholicity in the meal, not least in a culture in which access to food is "fenced". Jacobsen argues this requires a shift in eucharistic imagination from "private visions of 'family dinner' in favor of 'public banquet'" (Jacobsen 2018, p. 376). Granting the concerns documented by Jean Cotting about "entrapping" the "unbaptized in an unwanted obligation" (Cotting 2020, p. 234), the qualifying difference between the baptized and others gathered is that the former have a particular Christian appreciation of what God is doing in them. A less well-defined or simply different understanding brought by someone who does not share Christian faith need not mean exclusion from the symbol. On the contrary, it may contribute to the "surplus of meaning" that is the hallmark of liturgical prayer. To again invoke Carvalhaes, "if our worship space is really public, it means it will be a place where anyone can come and be a part of it" (Carvalhaes 2017, p. 284).

This inevitably leads to the adjournment of the assembly's gathering "until next time" presumably to embody in some form whatever new encounter with the living God it has experienced. While it may not be helpful to add more words to an already language-centric event, it would seem that an exit from the assembly must include a call to engage God's work in the world. Perhaps here the "business meeting" of the church might include an announcement of the "public service" it engages beyond the liturgy. It might also include those sent out immediately from the assembly to do the "liturgy after the liturgy" in the church's name, whether to carry food to relieve hunger or join others in common efforts to make public the "adjustment to deep change caused in the assembly by its being brought regularly to the brink of chaos in the presence of the living God," including engaging the risk this work might entail. As the assembly entered, so it goes out, as a body, to do the work the Spirit groans to have its members do. Moving through the liturgy together, as if in pilgrimage or even protest, might propose what Christopher Duraisingh has called the *concursus Dei*: "God's unceasing accompaniment with creation, calling and evoking [the assembly's] participation in God's movement as God leads it patiently and persuasively, both in judgment and grace, to its future in God's future" (Duraisingh 2010, p. 20).

5. Conclusion: Walking Together in Common Vulnerability

As I reflect on my own context, a church that shares a parking lot with a local hospital among the first to treat patients with COVID-19 in Illinois, I wish I had had the imagination to suggest that we take some of the risk asked of "essential workers": to gather in the safest way possible for a liturgy of pilgrimage around that hospital. Its "stations" might have refracted in lament, confession and prayer the risk borne by the "essential public service" of those caught between a natural pathogen and societal failure to engage it, as well as our own privileged "exemption" from that risk. I can imagine us calling the names of those bearing that risk—nurses' aides, food service workers, patients and their families—and inviting their prayers in conversation with hospital staff. Perhaps family members excluded from accompanying their loved ones might have joined us, enriching the symbol beyond our members and proposing a shared *koinonia* of common vulnerability to COVID-19. As that liturgy changed, it may have drawn greater attention to the injustices related to race, gender, and class unveiled and magnified over these many months and invited those gathered to action. We could not have saved anyone, but, as we surrounded and joined those most affected, we might have signified that *concursus Dei*, "mirroring the divine accompaniment through... solidarity and compassion with all" (Duraisingh 2010, p. 22).

29 "Open table" refers to practice in some Episcopal and other congregations that make an explicit invitation to all gathered to receive communion, regardless of whether they have been baptized or identify as Christian. This has been a subject of debate in my own Episcopal Church. See, for example, Cones (2016, pp. 693–96); and Malloy (2017, pp. 157–58).

Funding: This research received no external funding.

Conflicts of Interest: The author declares no conflict of interest.

References

Alexander, Neil M. 1992. *The United Methodist Book of Worship*. Nashville: The United Methodist Publishing House.
Anderson, Ron, Daniel Benedict, Gennifer Brooks, Dawn Chesser, Taylor Burton-Edwards, D. Stephen Long, L. Edward Philips, Don E. Saliers, and Karen Westerfield Tucker. 2020. Using Our Rites and Resources. Available online: https://www.ministrymatters.com/all/entry/10208/using-our-rites-and-resources (accessed on 21 December 2020).
Balasuriya, Tissa. 1977. *Eucharist and Human Liberation*. Sri Lanka: Centre for Society and Religion.
Belcher, Kimberly. 2020. Sacramental Exchange: Eschatological Economy and Consumption Ritual. *Religions* 11: 586. [CrossRef]
Bieler, Andrea, and Luise Schottroff. 2007. *The Eucharist: Bodies, Bread, and Resurrection*. Minneapolis: Fortress Press.
Bishops' Committee on the Liturgy. 1977. *Environment and Art in Catholic Worship*. Washington, DC: United States Catholic Conference.
Brown, Sally A. 2013. Discerning the Public Presence of God. *Theology Today* 70: 30–37. [CrossRef]
Burns, Stephen. 2020. Confessing More than Sin. In *When We Pray: The Future of Common Prayer*. Edited by Stephen Burns and Robert Gribben. Bayswater: Coventry Press, pp. 277–302.
Butler Bass, Diana. 2020. On Hoarding Eucharist in a Hungry World. Available online: https://churchanew.org/blog/posts/2020/05/01/butlerbass1 (accessed on 21 December 2020).
Carvalhaes, Cláudio. 2017. Worship, Liturgy and Public Witness. In *A Companion to Public Theology*. Edited by Kim Sebastian and Katie Day. Leiden: Brill, pp. 466–86. [CrossRef]
Carvalhaes, Cláudio. 2020. The Christian as *Humus*: Virtual/Real Earthly Rituals of Ourselves. *Liturgy* 35: 25–33. [CrossRef]
Cones, Bryan. 2016. The 78th General Convention of the Episcopal Church and the Liturgy: New Wine in Old Wineskins? *Anglican Theological Review* 98: 681–701.
Cones, Bryan. 2018. "Christ, Hear Us": The Assembly's Prayer for the World. *New Theology Review* 31: 69–71.
Cones, Bryan. 2020a. How Do We Gather Now? What We Have Lost—and Gained—through Virtual Worship. *The Christian Century* 137: 22–24, (26 August 2020). Available online: https://www.christiancentury.org/article/critical-essay/virtual-worship-has-become-people-s-work (accessed on 20 December 2020).
Cones, Bryan. 2020b. *This Assembly of Believers: The Gifts of Difference in the Church at Prayer*. London: SCM Press.
Copeland, M. Shawn. 2010. *Enfleshing Freedom: Body, Race, and Being*. Minneapolis: Fortress Press.
Cotting, Jean. 2020. Public Liturgy and Public Secularity: A Response to James W. Farwell. *Anglican Theological Review* 102: 231–34.
Curry, Michael. 2020. On Our Theology of Worship. Available online: https://episcopalchurch.org/posts/publicaffairs/presiding-bishop-michael-currys-word-church-our-theology-worship (accessed on 21 December 2020).
Duraisingh, Christopher. 2010. From Church-Shaped Mission to Mission-Shaped Church. *Anglican Theological Review* 92: 7–28.
Evangelical Lutheran Church in America. 2020. Worship in Times of Public Health Concerns: COVID-19/Coronavirus. Available online: https://download.elca.org/ELCA%20Resource%20Repository/Worship_in_Times_of_Public_Health_Concerns.pdf (accessed on 21 December 2019).
Farwell, James. 2020. Liturgy and Public Theology. *Anglican Theological Review* 102: 219–29.
Fennema, Sharon R. 2018. The Forgetfulness of Gentrification and the Pilgrimage of Protest: Re-Membering the Body of Christ. *Review & Expositor* 115: 378–85. [CrossRef]
Fensham, Charles James. 2016. The Transformative Vision: Public Witness and the Poiesis of Christian Social Transformation. *Missiology* 44: 155–66. [CrossRef]
Foley, Edward. 2008. Engaging the Liturgy of the World: Worship as Public Theology. *Studia Liturgica* 38: 31–52.
Graham, Elaine. 2020. Theology and the Public Square: Mapping the Field. *Modern Believing* 61: 7–21. [CrossRef]
Gribben, Robert. 2020. Eucharistic Absence. *Australian Journal of Liturgy* 17: 71–79.
Hellwig, Monika. 1992. *The Eucharist and the Hunger of the World*, 2nd ed. Revised and Expanded. Kansas City: Sheed & Ward.
Hovda, Robert. 1988. Celebrating Sacraments "For the Life of the World". *Worship* 62: 72–79.
Institute for Policy Studies. 2020a. COVID-19 and Inequality. Available online: https://inequality.org/facts/inequality-and-covid-19/ (accessed on 20 December 2020).
Institute for Policy Studies. 2020b. Updates: Billionaire Wealth, U.S. Job Losses and Pandemic Profiteers. Available online: https://inequality.org/great-divide/updates-billionaire-pandemic/ (accessed on 20 December 2020).
Jaycox, Michael P. 2017. Black Lives Matter and Catholic Whiteness: A Tale of Two Performances. *Horizons* 44: 306–41. [CrossRef]
Kavanagh, Aidan. 1984. *On Liturgical Theology*. New York: Pueblo Publishing Company.
Kubicki, Judith. 2006. *The Presence of Christ in the Gathered Assembly*. New York: Continuum.
Leatherland, Harold. 1974. Liturgy as Protest. *St. Mark's Review* 79: 17–22.
Lee, Jeffery D. 2020. Suspending In-Person Worship: A Letter from Bishop Lee. Available online: https://episcopalchicago.org/suspending-in-person-worship-a-letter-from-bishop-lee/ (accessed on 21 December 2020).
Malloy, Patrick L. 2017. The Principal Service Every Day: The Eucharist in Episcopal Life and the Weight of Revision. *Sewanee Theological Review* 61: 145–60.
Metropolitan Planning Council and Urban Institute. 2017. The Cost of Segregation: Lost Income. Lost Lives. Lost Potential. Available online: https://www.metroplanning.org/uploads/cms/documents/cost-of-segregation.pdf (accessed on 20 December 2020).

National Conference of State Legislatures. 2020. COVID-19: Essential Workers in the States. Available online: https://www.ncsl.org/research/labor-and-employment/covid-19-essential-workers-in-the-states.aspx (accessed on 21 December 2020).

Nóda, Mózes. 2017. Religion, Liturgy and Ethics, at the Intersection between Theory and Practice. The Revolution of Pope Francis. *Journal for the Study of Religion & Ideologies* 16: 17–33.

Rahner, Karl. 1976. Considerations on the Active Role of the Person in the Sacramental Event. In *Theological Investigations XIV*. Translated by David Bourke. New York: Seabury Press, pp. 161–84.

Ramshaw, Gail. 2017. *Pray, Praise, and Give Thanks: A Collection of Litanies, Laments, and Thanksgivings at the Font and Table*. Minneapolis: Augsburg Fortress.

Rhodes, Daniel. 2020. Life in the Struggle: Liturgical Innovation in the Face of the Cultural Devastation of Disaster Capitalism. *Journal of Moral Theology* 9: 94–114.

Rogers, Tiana N., Charles R. Rogers, Elizabeth VanSant-Webb, Lily Y. Gu, Bin Yan, and Fares Qeadan. 2020. Racial Disparities in COVID-19 Mortality Among Essential Workers in the United States. *World Medical & Health Policy* 12: 311–27. [CrossRef]

Sartore, Domenico. 1998. Pastoral Liturgy. In *Handbook for Liturgical Studies, vol. II: Fundamental Liturgy*. Edited by Anscar Chupungco. Collegeville: Liturgical Press, pp. 65–95.

Jacobsen, David Schnasa. 2018. Going Public with the Means of Grace: A Homiletical Theology of Promise for Word and Sacrament in a Post-Secular Age. *Theology Today* 75: 371–82. [CrossRef]

Scott, Emily M. D. 2020a. A Ritual to Honor Black Lives: Remembering People Killed by Police. *The Christian Century* 137: 30–33.

Scott, Hilton. 2020b. Worship in a Post-Lockdown Context: A Ritual-Liturgical Perspective. *HTS Teologiese Studies/Theological Studies* 76: 8. [CrossRef]

Searle, Mark. 1983. New Tasks, New Methods: The Emergence of Pastoral Liturgical Studies. *Worship* 57: 291–308.

Skelley, Michael. 1991. *The Liturgy of the World: Karl Rahner's Theology of Worship*. Collegeville: Liturgical Press.

Stewart, Benjamin M. 2012. Worship without Walls: Taking Liturgy to the Streets. *The Christian Century* 129: 22–25.

Suna-Koro, Kristine. 2019. Liturgy and Lament: Postcolonial Reflections from the Midst of a Global Refugee Crisis. *Liturgy* 34: 31–40. [CrossRef]

The Uniting Church in Australia. 2020. Temporary Arrangements for Holy Communion. Available online: https://uca.ut.je/cudw/worship-resources-and-publications/item/3033-temporary-arrangements-for-holy-communion (accessed on 21 December 2020).

Thompson, Deanna A. 2020. Christ Is Really Present, Even in Holy Communion via Online Worship. *Liturgy* 35: 18–24. [CrossRef]

religions

MDPI

Article

Liturgy in Lockdown: Restricted Movement, Expanded Worship

Deborah Ann Wong

Duke Divinity School, Duke University, Durham, NC 27708, USA; debbie.wong@duke.edu

Abstract: What has the pandemic taught us about worship? Reflecting on religion in quarantine, Heidi A. Campbell observed that while many churches have embraced a new medium of worship (digital), the underlying approach to worship has remained centered on the worship event. Campbell criticizes this event-based focus as being out of step with the networked age in which we live. Is Campbell right, or is there still a place for the worship event, even in this networked age? Drawing on the work of liturgical theologians and network theorists, I revisit the role of the liturgical event in the wider life of the church, arguing that the liturgical event remains a central element of the church's mission, but that the liturgy is meant to take worshippers beyond itself. I suggest that pandemic reflections on liturgy should lead the church to emphasize that Christians are a sent people, even during a time of restricted movement. This shift in emphasis from gathering to sending out redefines the church more broadly and helps us reclaim a more expansive vision of worship beyond the mere event.

Keywords: liturgy; worship; pandemic; network; liquid church; sacramentality

1. Introduction

In Season 2 Episode 1 of the BBC television adaptation, *Sherlock*, starring Benedict Cumberbatch, Sherlock Holmes employs a simple trick to discover the location of his nemesis Irene Adler's concealed safe: he has his colleague, John Watson, set off the fire alarm. As soon as the alarm goes off, Adler's eyes flicker toward the mirror behind which the safe is hidden, thus revealing its location. "Fire exposes our priorities," Holmes explains. Our instinct is to save the thing that we treasure most. Fire—or in our case, a global pandemic—reveals what we value most.

When the global pandemic hit North America in March 2020, businesses, schools, and churches alike were thrown into a state of literal emergency, forced to make quick decisions about how to continue their work in the midst of lockdowns and directives on social distancing. The urgency of the situation and the limitations imposed meant that leaders had to triage: What do we save first? On what should we focus our limited resources and energies? What must be preserved in order to ensure the continued existence of the church?

The answer for most churches, it seems, was worship—in particular, the worship service.

Analyzing the results of a two-part survey (MacDonald et al. 2020) of over 1500 pastors and leaders, conducted in March and April 2020, Heidi A. Campbell observed that pastors "overwhelmingly ranked conducting weekend services as their priority" (Campbell 2020, p. 10), whether that meant moving services online or doggedly insisting on meeting in person, despite government regulations and recommendations to the contrary. Campbell, who studies digital religion and new media, observes that this response reveals a primarily event-based understanding of religion that she argues is out of step with the networked age in which we live—one in which people experience community as a social network of relationships, rather than being centered around a single group, such as the church (Campbell 2020, p. 11).

Campbell is right to suggest that a Christian community that understands itself solely or even primarily in terms of its ability to gather together is missing a crucial element[1].

However, it is a different thing to suggest that this gathering is irrelevant to the networked age altogether. This dichotomy between an event-based and a networked approach to religious community is a false one, especially for the Christian community, which has always been both a networked community and one that gathers to worship. In this article, I try to nuance Campbell's argument by suggesting that the worship event remains a central element of the church's mission but it can properly occupy this center only as part of a broader mission that extends into a wider, ever-expanding network. The very telos of the worship gathering is the sending of people out into the vast networks of which they are a part, and within which they are encouraged to participate fully as disciples of Christ.

I begin by first exploring the arguments in support of the alternative that Campbell suggests—that of a networked model of religious community. I then consider a theological argument for the centrality of the worship event, asking whether the event and network approaches are truly dichotomous. Finally, I conclude by suggesting that what is needed is not a decentering of the worship event from the church community but rather a reclaiming of the event more fully, as one that is concerned with creating and sustaining a networked community that is both local and global, both situated and dispersed, both gathered and sent out.

2. Networked Religion: Beyond the Event

We live in a networked world. This claim has been made so often by now that it has become something of a cliché. To use another phrase that has recently suffered the same fate, this networked world is our "new normal", and has been for some time already. The idea of a networked society has been around since at least 1991, with the publication of Jan van Dijk's book *The Network Society* (van Dijk 1991), but Niall Ferguson argues that humans are in fact inherently oriented toward forming social networks and have always done so (Ferguson 2017). The sociologists Nicholas Christakis and James Fowler observe that "our brains seem to have been built for social networks" (Christakis and Fowler 2009, p. 239), and historians William H. McNeill and J.R. McNeill suggest that the "first worldwide web" in fact emerged about 12,000 years ago (McNeill and McNeill 2003, p. 4). This fact of life has simply been amplified and brought to the fore by what Lee Rainie and Barry Wellman referred to as the "triple revolution" of the internet, social media, and mobile networks (Rainie and Wellman 2012, pp. 11–20). Social media has simply made visible the networks of which we were already a part.

Among the features of what Rainie and Wellman call this "new social operating system" are a move away from a group or institutional identity, toward "networked individualism" and a corresponding shifting of authority structures (Rainie and Wellman 2012, p. 8). Whereas in the past, people's social networks used to be small and revolve tightly around family and community groups, they are now looser and more expansive. Where social relationships were once centered on these tightly knit groups, each individual is now the center of their own social network. With this shift comes a blurring of authority, as traditional hierarchies are diluted by the horizontal connections enabled by the social network. The Internet has made information that was once restricted to those with special expertise and training available to anyone with a smartphone who can spell "Wikipedia". Local pastors are no longer the only, or even the closest, spiritual authority to which individuals have access.

This shift in structure has been seen by some as a threat to the social fabric of society. In his study of America's declining social capital, Robert Putnam identified the shift away from group-based membership as a sign of the collapse of American community (Putnam 2000). Pastors and leaders of churches of all denominations, likewise, fear that the declining attendance at church services is a sign of decreased religiosity among their members. This focus on the number of worshipers in attendance is one of the negative outcomes that Campbell cites of an "event-based" approach to religious community (Campbell 2020). The assumption is that if people are not attending church, they are not engaging with or committed to their faith. With this approach, participation in the worship event is seen as the marker of one's religiosity and faithfulness.

While the reality of dwindling church attendance has led some pastors to double down on their efforts to make church services more engaging, in order to attract (and retain) members, a recognition of our networked reality has led others to adopt a different strategy. Instead of trying to bring people to church, they focus on bringing the church to where people already are. As early as 2002, Pete Ward began imagining what this might look like, expounding a vision of what he called the "liquid church" (Ward 2002). In contrast to a "solid church", which has at its center some form of congregational gathering (Campbell's "worship event"), a liquid church is fluid, taking its shape from the network of relationships that constitute it (Ward 2002, p. 48)[2]. In place of attending a weekly worship event, Ward suggests that the emphasis of a liquid church is "on living as Christ's body in the world" (Ward 2002, p. 2).

More recently, Keith Anderson has described this strategy in terms of a "digital cathedral," drawing on historic models of cathedrals that stood at the center of the city, in terms of both physical and social location (Anderson 2015). Like Ward's liquid church, Anderson writes that the "digital cathedral" is an invitation to "a more expansive understanding of church, and ways of being church, at a time when our definitions of church have become all too narrow, too parochial" (Anderson 2015, p. 20)—too "event-based," Campbell might say (Campbell 2020). Although much contemporary discussion (especially since the pandemic) has centered specifically on the church in relation to digital networks, Anderson notes that the idea of a digital cathedral is not solely a case of an online or digital church. Rather, this "networked, relational, and incarnational approach to ministry" urges church leaders to step out of the church and "be present in the places people work, live, and play," and to pay attention to the spirituality of everyday life, distinct from "the formal spirituality of the institutional church" (Anderson 2015, p. 30).

Anderson tells of ministry initiatives ranging from theology pub gatherings to Bible studies held in coffee shops, to handing out coffee and donuts on a street corner, as examples of this way of living "in cathedral" (Anderson 2015, p. 8). Each of these initiatives represents an attentiveness to the spirituality of everyday life—what Jeanne Halgren Kilde describes as a "situational" approach to sacred space, in which sacred space is constructed by the actions and meanings that humans assign to it. This stands in contrast to a "substantive" approach, which limits sacred space to designated "religious" places like churches (Kilde 2008). The situational approach, represented by Ward's liquid church and Anderson's digital cathedral, expands the religious community beyond the church building by recognizing ordinary places as sacred too. Reflecting the features of our networked age, it decenters the traditional hierarchical structure that constrained the religious community within the church's walls, creating space to acknowledge that there are other ways to engage faithfully in religious community outside of participation in the worship event.

However, this raises a key ecclesiological question: Is participation in a worship service equivalent to participation in any gathering of Christians? Are theology pub gatherings to be considered a substitute for participation in the liturgy, or is there something about the formal liturgical event that still warrants a significant place in churches' understanding of religious community? Put differently, is it enough simply that we gather, or do how we gather and what we do when we gather also make a difference? Is there still a place for the worship event in this networked, liquid age?

3. What Is at Stake in the Worship Event?

Those who advocate a networked approach to religion point to the fact that God is present everywhere, not limited by time or space, that God is not limited to the church, that everyday ordinary places can themselves be imbued with sacred significance and likewise be places where one might encounter God—and they are surely correct. Yet all around the world, Christians continue to meet to worship together. Is this simply, as Campbell suggests, a failure to adapt to the reality of the networked age? Or is there something about the worship event that remains valuable, even in this liquidized and networked age?

The pastors in the survey that Campbell analyzed evidently believe that the worship event continues to hold a place of importance in the Christian life, and they are not alone in thinking so. The Church has traditionally heeded the exhortation of the writer of the letter to the Hebrews to not neglect meeting together (Hebrews 10: v. 25) as a divine injunction to gather regularly in worship[3]. But what is it that we do in worship that makes it so important? Or, perhaps, the better question is: what is it that worship does to us?

Firstly, worship forms us. Liturgical theologians speak of the liturgy as being "formal," which is to say that it has the capacity to create form—to shape those who participate in it (Fagerberg 2011). Aidan Kavanagh is reported to have often remarked, "I don't go to Mass because I'm Catholic, I'm Catholic because I go to Mass". The liturgy, enacted in the worship event, is not simply about Christians gathering—it is an important factor in what forms them into Christians in the first place. In the worship event, God acts through the liturgy to shape us into God's people, a people who, among other things, are able to recognize God's presence and work in the world, and to see all of creation as sacred.

The everyday spirituality for which network models of religious community call requires a sacramental vision that does not come naturally to fallen, sinful humans. As Alexander Schmemann argues, however, the true reality of the world is that it is "shot through with the presence of God", although we may often fail to see it as such (Schmemman 2018, p. 17). This sacramental approach to the world *is*, in fact, the natural way in which Christians ought to experience the world, but in order to do so, our vision must be renewed such that we, in St. Ignatius of Loyola's words, might "see God in all things". What we do in the worship event forms in us this capacity to see sacramentally—in St. Augustine's terms, to see one thing, yet perceive another (Augustine 1993).

The "official" sacraments, whether seven or two or another number, are clear places where we learn this sacramental vision. In the waters of baptism, and the bread and wine of the Eucharist, we learn that ordinary things can be vehicles for the extraordinary (Schmemman would say that it is the "extraordinary" that is, in fact, ordinary in the true reality of God's kingdom). Similarly, Thomas Groome writes that "the great sacraments are simply climactic celebrations of the sacramentality of life" (Groome 2012), intensifications of the general sacramentality that can be found in the world. Yet, even churches that do not have the sacraments at the center of their worship each week offer opportunities to be trained in this sacramental vision. The very assertion that the church is the body of Christ requires the ability to perceive a spiritual reality beyond the physical. How else are we to believe that these people with whom we have gathered—some of whom may, in fact, be strangers to us, others with whom we would like to have nothing to do—are related to us by a bond that is stronger and more binding than the blood that ties us to our earthly families? What is more, how else are we to believe that this ragtag bunch of people are somehow the embodiment of Christ on this earth?

The proper focus of the worship event, then, is not mere attendance but transformation, with an eye toward daily Christian living. The philosopher James K.A. Smith reminds us that the "formal" nature of liturgy is not limited to Christian worship. Smith asserts that we are constantly being formed by the practices and liturgies in which we participate, including cultural and "secular" practices that are as seemingly mundane as a shopping trip to the mall (Smith 2009). In particular, Smith argues that our actions are governed by desire, and it is our desires that are subject to this formation (and malformation) (Smith 2009, p. 53)[4]. All liturgies promote a certain vision of the good life and shape our desires accordingly. The worship event is thus critically important because it serves as "a counter-formation to the mis-formation of secular liturgies into which we are 'thrown' from an early age" (Smith 2009, p. 88). Not only does it renew our vision, so that we are able to see all of creation as sacraments of God's grace but it also forms in us the desire to bear witness to God's grace in the world as the body of Christ, ourselves becoming signs of God's grace. Participating in the Christian worship event also shapes us to be the kind of people who *desire* to fulfill the goals of Ward's liquid church, Anderson's digital cathedral, and other networked approaches to church and religion—namely, to "[live] as Christ's body in the world" (Ward 2002, p. 2).

This leads to a second, related point: in the worship event, we are commissioned for this very thing: to be the body of Christ in the world. The worship event does not end with us simply leaving because the event is over. Rather, having been transformed through our encounter with Christ in worship, we are *sent* out—*commissioned*—to "be for the world the body of Christ," as the United Methodist Communion liturgy states. In his forthcoming book, Edward Foley makes a compelling case that the Eucharistic liturgy of the Catholic church is essentially an amplification of the Great Commission to "go forth and make disciples of all nations" (Matthew 28: v. 19) (Foley Forthcoming). Yet, again, even in the absence of the Lord's Supper in a worship service, Constance Cherry (2012) writes that the worship event most appropriately finishes with a blessing and a charge (commission), such as, "Go in peace (blessing) to love and serve the Lord (charge)". The "end" of worship is the "beginning" of mission; but, more accurately, they are one and the same.

In gathered worship, we are constituted as the body of Christ, the church. Inherent in this constitution is a responsibility to continue God's mission, Christ's work on earth. While Jesus walked the earth, anyone wanting to receive a blessing could simply approach him. Crowds came from miles away to listen to him speak words of life. When a man needed healing, he waited for Christ to pass by and cried out, "Son of David, have mercy on me!" The blind man asked to see, and Jesus spat on the ground and rubbed the mud on his eyes. While Jesus walked the earth, it was obvious where you needed to be if you needed something only Christ could give. Since the Ascension, however, Jesus is no longer physically on earth. How, then, can anyone receive healing, salvation, forgiveness, or grace from the Lord? Who will do the Father's work, now that Christ is no longer physically present for the world to interact with[5]? Karl Rahner asserts that "[the church] is the primary sacrament through which Christ manifests and effects his saving grace in the world" (Skelley 1991, p. 156). If the Church takes seriously the proposition that she is now the body of Christ in the world, and the means through which Christ communicates his grace, the Church must always fulfill its mission in and to the world to proclaim good news to the poor, bind up the brokenhearted, proclaim freedom for the captives, care for the widows and orphans, and look after the least of these.

The incarnational ministry that appeals to proponents of networked religion is, thus, most properly understood as the natural outcome of the church at worship—the way the church fulfills its commission. Far from being at odds with one another, the worship event and the network model are two sides of the same coin. The worship event is never to be seen as self-contained, but as having a telos that is aimed outward, sending the people of God forth into the world, with the ability to witness to the work of God in everyday life as they live in networked community with others. Failure to attend to this telos results, as Campbell rightly observes, in too narrow an understanding of religious community—as well as too narrow a view of the worship event (whether online or in person). If the worship event is seen as an end in itself, its telos remains unfulfilled. Fagerberg speaks of the worship event as merely the "tip of the liturgical iceberg," the part visible above water (Fagerberg 2011). This image reinforces the idea that although the event is seen to be central to Christian community, it does not—and cannot—exist in isolation. Furthermore, to focus only on the tip of the liturgical iceberg is to fall prey to what Paul Holmer terms "liturgical hyperconsciousness," becoming overly conscious and enamored of the liturgy rather than allowing the liturgy to make us conscious of God, and the mission of God in which God has called us to participate (Holmer 1976, p. 24). Conversely, an overemphasis on the "mission" without the worship risks reducing that missionary work in networks to little more than human activity. The missiologist David Bosch reminds us that the church engages in mission not chiefly as a work of its own but in order to be a reflection of Christ in the world (Bosch 1991)[6]. That is, being missional is simply part of who God is, and thus by extension, who the church ought to be. The mission belongs to and begins with

God, not the church. In worship, the Church receives her commission to participate in this mission of God. Far from narrowing the definition of religious community, then, a proper understanding of the worship event as being inextricably linked through mission to the worshipers' networked reality results in the possibility of an ever-expanding religious community—one that spreads out in the form of a network but that is gathered at and by a central hub.

4. Conclusions

The idea I have put forth here, that the church's worship life extends beyond the worship event, is not a novel one. It has, however, at times been obscured or forgotten, resulting in a division between what many have referred to as the church's gathered worship and scattered worship[7]. The church *gathers* to worship (in the "worship event") and then *scatters* to live out God's mission in the world through networks of which the worshipers are a part. Both are an integral part of what it means to worship, and thus the worship event cannot be seen as an outdated model of the church's life together—it is merely an incomplete one. Even in his proposal of a liquid church model, Pete Ward acknowledged that "worship and meeting with others will still have a place" (Ward 2002, p. 2). Both Ward's (2002) and Anderson's (2015) underlying concerns about the established church seem not to be with a sense of its outdatedness, but with its insularity and narrowness in terms of effectively confining God to the church building or worship event. That is, what is "out of step with the networked age" (Campbell 2020) is not the fact that the church meets to worship together but that it expects this event to be the primary mode of mission. Sadly, the modern church has, indeed, often prioritized the gathering to the exclusion of the sending. However, the solution is not to do away with the gathering but to reclaim it in its entirety—as the hub that centrifugally powers the many nodes linked to it in the larger network.

What does all this mean for the liturgy in the midst of a pandemic? First, I believe it affirms the instincts of those pastors and leaders who focused on trying to maintain a worship gathering. At the same time, however, it reminds us that the goal of these offerings is not simply to reach a certain level of viewership or attendance. Understandably, many pastors lament the lower viewership for their online services, compared to in-person attendees, fearing that their congregants are no longer engaging in religious community. The fear is a valid one, but an expansive, outward-facing understanding of the worship event reminds us that viewership numbers might not be the best metric to focus on, whether in terms of accuracy or mission. Instead, a properly balanced approach that recognizes the telos of the event to be the commissioning of its participants "to be for the world the body of Christ" should have as one of its main goals the equipping of the people being sent forth.

In any case, anecdotal evidence suggests that while some have indeed stopped going to church altogether and have not engaged in alternative forms of religious activity, many others have found new ways of worshiping through the practices of morning and evening prayer, liturgies written for "the ordinary events of daily life"[8], and various online religious communities on social media. They have found ways to live in the sacramentality of everyday life, knowing that God's gifts of grace are not out of reach. Thus, the fearful conclusion that congregants who are not attending services online have forsaken worship practices altogether may not be entirely true.

In cases where it *is* true, what should trouble pastors most is not the fact that these congregants are not attending church but that their previous participation in worship has not formed them into a people whose worship continues even beyond and in the absence of the worship event[9]. This should be a concern even during non-pandemic times, but just as the pandemic reveals our priorities, it exposes our vulnerabilities and draws our attention to areas that may have otherwise been neglected. The role of the worship event has not changed as a result of the pandemic, but, in the wake of COVID-19, online church services, and incredible Zoom fatigue, some churches may find that they have been guilty of a kind of "liturgical hyperconsciousness" (Holmer 1976, p. 24), concerned more about the execution of the liturgical event than its formative power. A crucial question that the pandemic should be leading church leaders to ask, then, is: How is the way that we conduct worship forming, or failing to form, in parishioners the capacity to approach sacred space situationally, to see in every place, person and ritual the possibility of an encounter with the living God?

Perhaps more specifically, how do we teach and encourage parishioners to pay attention to the spirituality of everyday life, such that, even in the absence of regular weekly gatherings, they might continue to recall the life, death and resurrection of Christ and live accordingly as faithful disciples of Christ? How do we help parishioners to understand the mission with which they are sent forth from the worship event into the world, especially at a time when the world into which they are sent forth is one largely confined within the walls of their home? What resources are we providing or failing to provide for parishioners to equip them to develop these capacities? Furthermore, with many churches planning to continue meeting online beyond the end of the pandemic, more creative attention needs to be given to how this formation can best be facilitated through both online and offline mediums. As media theorists have long insisted, the medium is not neutral, and different mediums (and contexts) require different approaches to the same issue. What works for an in-person assembly will almost certainly differ from what works best for an online assembly[10].

I have suggested that the worship event, properly conceived, is intended to point worshipers beyond the event (and themselves), that the directionality of its telos is outward, into the world (both physical and virtual). Having encountered Christ, His disciples were sent into the world with the promise that Christ would be with them always, and with an accompanying charge to make other disciples (Matthew 28: vv. 19–20). Rather than keeping worshipers captive to itself, the liturgy (by facilitating an encounter with the risen Christ) similarly sends us forth into the world and frees us to discern the light of Christ and the work of the Spirit more fully in the world at large. This enables worshipers to both appreciate and participate in the sacramentality of ordinary, everyday life, and to *be* for the world a kind of sacrament through which they might experience and encounter the grace of God. In this regard, although the pandemic has shaken the foundations of many churches' worship life in numerous ways, Christian communities might view it not as a restriction on their worship, but rather as an invitation to reclaim a more expansive vision of worship that begins in the event but continues far beyond it, inviting us to encounter and serve God everywhere and at all times—even in the midst of a global pandemic.

Funding: This research received no external funding.

Institutional Review Board Statement: Not applicable.

Informed Consent Statement: Not applicable.

Data Availability Statement: Not applicable.

Conflicts of Interest: The author declares no conflict of interest.

Notes

1 A crucial question the pandemic forced churches to wrestle with is that of whether a *physical, in-person* gathering is a crucial component of the church's identity, or if a virtual, online gathering can be considered equally legitimate. Along with scholars such as Berger (2017), Drescher (2011), Thompson (2016), Gorrell (2019) and others, this author affirms the basic legitimacy of online worship in terms of Christ's ability to be present online, and the possibility of meaningful connection with God and others. At the same time, I acknowledge that not all forms or practices of online worship are equal or equivalent (just as not all forms or practices of in-person worship are equal or equivalent), and that the medium itself does not guarantee any specific outcomes (see notes 3 and 10 for further discussion). Regardless of one's opinions on the matter, however, online worship is a given of our present and future age. The task at hand is to figure out how to do it *well* (and, indeed, what it means to worship well). Thus, rather than addressing the online versus in-person worship debate in detail (which would require an entirely separate article or series of articles in itself), the present article seeks to engage what I consider to be an even more foundational question, regarding the relationship between the Church's worship event and her participation in God's mission. The temptation and danger of

seeing these elements as separate or separable is common to both online and in-person gatherings, and my contention here is that a clear vision of worship itself as part of this missionary endeavor must precede any strategies related to the technicalities of the gathering, whether in person or online.

2 Ward borrows the language of "solid" and "liquid" from the Polish philosopher and sociologist Zygmunt Bauman, who distinguishes between solid and liquid modernity. Bauman (2000) argued that modernity was in the process of being liquidized, such that individuals can no longer base their identity on organizations or institutions but must instead shape their identity through their own choices. Ward observes that whereas solid modernity spawned a solid form of church, the liquid modernity of the present demands a liquid form of church. For our purposes, we can consider this liquidized society synonymous with the networked age that we have been discussing.

3 Proponents of what Jay Kim (2020) calls the "analog church" argue that the kind of gathering that the writer of the letter to the Hebrews has in mind is an in-person one. They point to the Incarnation's implication of bodily significance and insist that Christian worship must take place in person if it is to avoid a Gnosticism that renders our physical bodies insignificant. The liturgical historian Andrew McGowan (2020) notes that Christian worship has generally implied a community that is physically present in one place. In response, advocates of online worship take the view expressed by Lawrence Lessig in his "The Zones of Cyberspace" (Lessig 1996) that "Cyberspace is a place. People live there". Incarnational living thus extends to cyberspace, which is no less *real*, although it may be virtual. Online worship is not, or at least need not be a disembodied experience. Cyberspace is, thus, seen as a new mission field in its own right, inviting the Church to extend Christ's ministry and presence to the ends of the internet. Surely, even there, Christ will be with them by the power of the Spirit. Of course, there is much more to be said about this debate. As mentioned earlier, however, I believe the conversation must move beyond a debate about the basic validity of online worship and focus instead on its potential for both formation and malformation, as well as what full, conscious, and active participation in online worship might look like. (Indeed, a renewed focus on these dynamics in in-person worship services is also needed!)

4 Key to Smith's argument is a theological anthropology that views humans as creatures of desire. Subverting the Cartesian notion that we are what we think, which has largely dominated Protestantism at least since the Reformation, Smith takes a more Augustinian view that humans are what we *love*. Thus, worship is one of the means through which we are taught to love rightly.

5 I am indebted to the liturgical historian Lester Ruth for this insight.

6 I am grateful to Edward Foley for introducing me to Bosch's work, and to the maxim that it is not that the church has a mission, but that God's mission has a church.

7 See, for example, a recent (modified) use of this phrase in (Hudson 2019). Hudson's argument is similar to mine: he argues that what the church does on Sunday ought to "empower people to live faithfully and fruitfully for Christ in their Monday-to-Saturday lives".

8 See, for example: (McKelvey 2017) and (McKelvey 2021), (Stokes 2021), and (Bevins 2020).

9 This is what Karl Rahner refers to as "the liturgy of the world," which he views as having priority over "the liturgy of the church". In the framework I have laid out here, we might explain this priority in this way: our worship in church is meaningless if it does not lead to our worship being lived out in the world.

10 The theologian Deanna Thompson (2016) tells of her own conversion from a "digital skeptic" to a firm believer in the power and potential of virtual connectedness as a result of being bed-bound by cancer and, thus, being forced to rely on virtual means of finding and sustaining community. She is quick to point out, however, that digital technology itself does not guarantee community. Felicia Wu Song (2009) makes a similar observation, in *Virtual Communities: Bowling Alone, Online Together*, that virtual communities do not automatically introduce a new dynamic of community but in fact reinforce existing assumptions about the self and community. Along with Thompson, I believe that technology is best seen as a tool that complements and extends God's mission, as expressed in physical congregations to online spaces, and more attention needs to be paid to the unique gifts that various forms of technology bring to the table. I think the question of whether online worship can fully replace in-person worship is useful only insofar as it functions as a thought experiment to help us identify core liturgical concerns. The reality is that online worship is happening, for better and for worse. Each mode of worship, both analog and digital, offers different gifts to and through the church. A disembodied theoretical discussion about the superiority and inferiority of these modes ignores the local and specific contexts and the needs of individual congregations and congregants. What is clear from the last year and a half is that some people have found greater connection and meaning through worshiping online, while others have found themselves utterly unable to do so. Many who, because of illness, social anxiety, work, or a variety of other factors, would not otherwise step foot inside a church for worship have become faithful congregants online, while others who are unable to engage online have stopped attending worship altogether. My hope is that this discussion helps to facilitate a shift from a narrow debate between the absolute validity and superiority of an online or offline church to imaginative conversations about liturgical robustness and formation in a universal church that extends throughout the physical and virtual world.

References

Anderson, Keith. 2015. *The Digital Cathedral: Networked Ministry in a Wired World*. New York: Morehouse Publishing.

Augustine, Saint. 1993. Sermon 272. In *Sermons:(230-272B) on the Liturgical Seasons, vol. III/7*. Edited by John E. Rotelle. Translated by O. P. Ed-Mund Hill. New York: New City Press.

Bauman, Zygmunt. 2000. *Liquid Modernity*. Cambridge: Polity Press.
Berger, Teresa. 2017. *@Worship: Liturgical Practices in Digital Worlds*. New York: Routledge.
Bevins, Winfield. 2020. *Living Room Liturgy*. Franklin: Seedbed Publishing.
Bosch, David J. 1991. *Transforming Mission: Paradigm Shifts in Theology of Mission*. New York: Orbis Books.
Campbell, Heidi A. 2020. Religion Embracing and Resisting Cultural Change in a Time of Social Distancing. In *Religion in Quarantine: The Future of Religion in a Post-Pandemic World*. Edited by Heidi A. Campbell. College Station: Digital Religion Publications, Available online: https://hdl.handle.net/1969.1/188004 (accessed on 17 November 2020).
Cherry, Constance. 2012. *The Worship Architect: A Blueprint for Designing Culturally Relevant and Biblically Faithful Services*. Grand Rapids: Baker Academic.
Christakis, Nicholas A., and James H. Fowler. 2009. *Connected: The Surprising Power of Our Social Networks and How They Shape Our Lives*. New York: Little, Brown.
Drescher, Elizabeth. 2011. *Tweet if You [Heart] Jesus: Practicing Church in a Digital Reformation*. Harrisburg: Morehouse Pub.
Fagerberg, David W. 2011. Being formed into liturgical people by an abiding *lex orandi*. Paper presented at Southwest Liturgical Conference, Salt Lake City, UT, USA, February 3.
Ferguson, Niall. 2017. *The Square and the Tower: Networks, Hierarchies, and the Struggle for Global Power*. London: Penguin Books.
Foley, Edward. Forthcoming. *Eucharistic Adoration after Vatican II*. Collegeville: Liturgical Press.
Gorrell, Angela. 2019. *Always On: Practicing Faith in a New Media Landscape*. Grand Rapids: Baker Academic.
Groome, Thomas H. 2012. What Makes Us Catholic: The Sacramental Principle. In *C21 Resources*. Boston: The Church in the 21st Century, Boston College, pp. 4–5.
Holmer, Paul. 1976. About Liturgy and Its Logic. *Worship* 50: 18–28.
Hudson, Neil. 2019. *Scattered and Gathered: Equipping Disciples for the Frontline*. London: Intervarsity Press.
Kilde, Jeanne Halgren. 2008. *Sacred Power, Sacred Space: An Introduction to Christian Architecture and Worship*. Oxford: Oxford University Press.
Kim, Jay. 2020. *Analog Church: Why We Need Real People, Places, and Things in the Digital Age*. Downers Grove: InterVarsity Press.
Lessig, Lawrence. 1996. The Zones of Cyberspace. *Stanford Law Review* 48: 1403–11. [CrossRef]
MacDonald, Andrew, Ed Stetzer, and Todd Wilson. 2020. How Church Leaders Are Responding to the Challenge of COVID-19. COVID-19 Church Survey Summary Report. Exponential. Available online: https://exponential.org/resource-ebooks/response-to-covid-19 (accessed on 10 November 2020).
McGowan, Andrew. 2020. Liturgy in a Time of Plague: A Letter to a Colleague. *Blog Post*. March 14. Available online: http://abmcg.blogspot.com/2020/03/liturgy-in-time-of-plague.html (accessed on 14 December 2021).
McKelvey, Douglas. 2017. *Every Moment Holy*. Nashville: Rabbit Room Press, vol. 1.
McKelvey, Douglas. 2021. *Every Moment Holy*. Nashville: Rabbit Room Press, vol. 2.
McNeill, John Robert, and William H. McNeill. 2003. *The Human Web: A Bird's-Eye View of World History*. New York: W.W. Norton & Company.
Putnam, Robert. 2000. *Bowling Alone: The Collapse and Revival of American Community*. New York: Simon & Schuster.
Rainie, Lee, and Barry Wellman. 2012. *Networked: The New Social Operating System*. Cambridge: MIT Press.
Schmemman, Alexander. 2018. *For the Life of the World: Sacraments and Orthodoxy*. Yonkers: St Vladimir's Seminary Press.
Skelley, Michael S. J. 1991. *The Liturgy of the World: Karl Rahner's Theology of Worship*. Collegeville: Liturgical Press.
Smith, James K. A. 2009. *Desiring the Kingdom: Worship, Worldview, and Cultural Formation*. Grand Rapids: BakerAcademic.
Stokes, Terry J. 2021. *Prayers for the People: Things We Didn't Know We Could Say to God*. New York: Convergent Books.
Thompson, Deanna A. 2016. *The Virtual Body of Christ in a Suffering World*. Nashville: Abingdon Press.
van Dijk, Jan A. G. M. 1991. *De Netwerkmaatschappij: Sociale Aspecten Van Nieuwe Media*, 1st ed. Houten: Bohn Staflen van Loghum.
Ward, Pete. 2002. *Liquid Church: A Bold Vision of How to Be God's People in Worship and Mission—A Flexible, Fluid Way of Being Church*. Peabody: Hendrickson Publishers, Inc.
Wu Song, Felicia. 2009. *Virtual Communities: Bowling Alone, Online Together*. New York: Peter Lang Publishing.

religions

MDPI

Article

"It's Your Breath in Our Lungs": Sean Feucht's Praise and Worship Music Protests and the Theological Problem of Pandemic Response in the U.S.

Adam A. Perez

Duke University Divinity School, Durham, NC 27712, USA; adam.perez@duke.edu

Abstract: In response to U.S. government restrictions imposed as part of a nationwide response to the COVID-19 pandemic, charismatic worship leader Sean Feucht began a series of worship concerts. Feucht positioned these protests as expressions of Christian religious freedom in opposition to mandated church closings and a perceived double-standard regarding the large gatherings of protesters over police violence against Black and Brown persons. Government restrictions challenged the sine qua non liturgical act of encounter with God for evangelicals, Pentecostals, and Charismatics: congregational singing in Praise and Worship. However, as Feucht's itinerant worship concerts traversed urban spaces across the U.S. to protest these restrictions, the events gained a double valence. Feucht and event attendees sought to channel God's power through musical worship to overturn government mandates and, along the way, they invoked longstanding social and racial prejudices toward urban spaces. In this essay, I argue that Feucht's events reveal complex theological motivations that weave together liturgical-theological, social, and political concerns. Deciphering this complex tapestry requires a review of both the history of evangelical engagement with urban spaces and the theological history of Praise and Worship. Together, these two sets of historical resources generate a useful frame for considering how Feucht, as a charismatic musical worship leader, attempts to wield spiritual power through musical praise to change political situations and the social conditions.

Keywords: Praise and Worship; praise; Sean Feucht; Pentecostal worship; pandemic; COVID-19; political theology

1. Introduction

Since midsummer 2020, contemporary praise and worship music leader Sean Feucht has been making news headlines for a series of public worship events held in cities across the U.S. He has branded the events by fusing religious and political language under the social media-friendly hashtag #letusworship. These public, ad-hoc, contemporary praise and worship music events in cities across the U.S. have also provided the occasion for Feucht's live worship music recordings, social media posts, and the sale of various kinds of merchandise.[1] His efforts have been met with strong praise by some (including by some from Bill Johnson's Bethel Church, a prominent megachurch in Redding, CA with which he has been affiliated) and deep ire by other Christians and by public officials. Given these religious affiliations and connections, it is somewhat surprising that the media coverage and public discourse around Feucht's events have not considered the worship theology of Praise and Worship as a primary motivating factor. When viewed through the lens of Praise and Worship liturgical theology, the problem that pandemic closures and public protests pose for Pentecostals—and other Praise and Worship practitioners among Charismatic and Evangelical Christians (Ingalls 2018)—comes into clearer focus.

Feucht has billed the events as a Christian response to the "spirit of fear" that has caused many churches to temporarily shut their doors. The events are also an avenue for Pentecostal, Charismatic, and Evangelical Christians[2] to publicly voice and embody their dissent to the perceived targeting and silencing of Christian religious freedom through COVID19-related government ordinances. Feucht's website describes the impetus for the movement, saying,

> The fervor to worship God free from government edict and societal persecution drove America's earliest settlers across oceans and wild frontiers. But our freedom to worship God and obey His Word has come under unprecedented attack. Powerful politicians and social media giants have engaged in unchartered abuses of religious liberty, silencing the faithful, banning our voices, and outright attacking our God-given right to declare His goodness. States across America, including right here in California, have shut down church services and even outlawed singing in church. It's time for the Church to rise up with one voice and tell our government leaders and the rulers of big tech that we refuse to be silenced! ("Let Us Worship" n.d.)

To that end, many of his events have been hosted at or near official public buildings (such as the Nashville Courthouse) or the sites of prominent U.S. monuments (such as on the Washington Mall). The political element of his protests is an especially salient feature for Feucht in his home state of California, where he lost a campaign bid for the 3rd congressional district in March 2020 a campaign expressly aimed at combatting the actions of Democratic Gov. Gavin Newsom.[3] His first #letusworship events began just a few months after his failed campaign. Though some of his events have skirted public health guidelines and local permit requirements, he has highlighted public baptisms as markers of God's blessing on the events such his New Year's Eve 2020 event on Skid Row in Los Angeles (Mayfield 2020; Spera 2020; Duin 2020).[4] All the while, Feucht has continued to build a digital brand, social media presence, and commercial success in the overlapping communities of American Evangelicals, anti-mask proponents, and #AllLivesMatter pundits.

This essay explores the question of why a Pentecostal musical worship leader has joined the national political conflict over mask mandates and limitations on public gatherings through worship music gatherings. I suggest that the answer to that question cannot be found solely in sociological descriptions of Pentecostals and their political preferences. It is not simply in counter-protests and public speeches that this community of Christians has responded to the pandemic crises. Instead, I propose that understanding Sean Feucht's worship protest events requires insight into the theology of Praise and Worship as a liturgical phenomenon. In looking to the theology of Praise and Worship, we see that music is not incidental to the protests but is part of a theological vision for responding to the present national crises.

I begin by addressing the recent historical context of urban engagement among Pentecostals, treating Pentecostals under the larger "evangelical" umbrella. This discussion is necessary for understanding the complexity of missional attitudes among evangelicals toward the urban settings where Feucht's events have been held, including Washington D.C. I also review the ways liturgical studies has traditionally considered the relationship between public liturgical gatherings and urban spaces and I suggest that these well-worn paths are perhaps insufficient for understanding contemporary instantiations of urban public worship rituals among Pentecostals and evangelicals. Turning to the core of the essay, I describe how historical sources in the development of Praise and Worship theology can illuminate our understanding of the significance of Feucht's public gatherings for those gathered. In making this connection, I show how the theology of music in worship is operationalized toward apparent political ends ways and is not merely incidental to the broader connection between political views and evangelical worship practices. Doing so suggests that the theology of Praise and Worship music is a particularly important driving force and avenue for political and social engagement among Pentecostals.

2. Evangelical Urban Engagement

The setting of urban spaces as sites for theological and political contestation via worship is not new to liturgical history. The academic study of the intersection between public worship and urban spaces has often focused on stational liturgies and the relationship between local churches as they become sites for city-wide processional celebrations on important feast days. John Baldovin's work on stational liturgies in Rome illuminates the way stational liturgies have functioned to demonstrate (and enact) the social and political legitimacy of Christianity within major urban centers of regional political power (Baldovin 1987).

However, the kinship between the political and the liturgical in urban spaces takes on an entirely new dimension in the late twentieth and early twenty first centuries. Before discussing more recent examples, it is important to briefly situate acts of public worship within the broader discourse of evangelical postures toward urban settings.

Evangelicalism (and its worship) has had a unique relationship with urban spaces. For evangelicals, urban spaces have been centers for the large evangelistic events and revivals that have come to characterize the tradition as a whole. In an essay on the multifarious ways conservative white Evangelicals have related to the city over the last century, Elisha summarizes this evangelical posture saying,

> [C]ities are stages—literally and figuratively—from which the Christian gospel of sin and redemption can be proclaimed to national and global audiences, and the tenets of conservative Protestantism projected upon secular society. As a result of these ambiguities, contemporary white evangelicals tend to regard the city as both Devil's playground and a key battleground in their struggles for cultural hegemony. For popular revivalists like Billy Graham, and influential parachurch organizations like the Promise Keepers, the great American city provides an ideal space for massive spectacles of public religiosity and the formation of powerful institutional networks which are used to revitalize the spiritual climate of the entire nation. (Omri 2010, pp. 235–36)

In this way, Feucht's narrative of nationwide revival through itinerant worship-evangelism events is hardly unique in their positioning or their aspirations. As Emily Snider Andrews has noted, "Renewalist" evangelicals like Bethel Church (and its affiliates like Feucht) actively attempt to instantiate a "kingdom culture" in the world through their daily lives (Snider Andrews 2020). Indeed, quoting Elisha again, "Their moral ambitions are infused with the spiritual and cultural aspirations of transforming urban social and institutional networks so that the values that become dominant are in accordance with the principles of God's kingdom" (Omri 2010, p. 236) Related rhetoric around this issue has also tended toward militant language of (spiritual) warfare for God's kingdom (Payne 2021). As we will see, public musical worship gatherings are, for this new era of Praise and Worship, an extension of a similar process of extending spiritual and political influence.

Of course, the religious and political conflicts over COVID-19 were not the only features of public discourse in mid-2020. The early summer saw a groundswell of activism in response to the murder of George Floyd by Minneapolis police officer Derek Chauvin. It was a flashpoint in the uproar related to other contemporaneous, police-involved shootings of Black and African American persons across the U.S. Just as churches were being told to cease indoor public worship services because of COVID-19 concerns, outdoor gatherings for protests over racism were ramping up and were (mostly) not prohibited by government officials. It is important to note here that for many evangelical political conservatives, protests and protesters are generally viewed with an air of suspicion. Add to that the problematic fact that these were protests against police officers, a class of service persons who have long been heralded in public discourse as heroes of American (Christian) society (Du Mez 2020). Thus the particular relationship to the city is marked both by evangelistic efforts that assume a spiritual depravity of urban spaces (i.e., a "Devil's playground") and, as a result of the processes of "white flight" from urban spaces into the suburbs since the 1950s, also encodes a racial dynamic into the pandemic tension (Mulder 2015).

In effect, multiple layers of the politics of race and religion created a strong cocktail of white American Christian nationalism that have fueled national debates over governance. To many politically conservative Christians (often generalized in media outlets as the monolith of "American Evangelicals"), the comparison of limitations on public worship versus the freedom of public protest were portrayed as a prejudicial incongruence against Christians and the practice of the freedom of Christian religion in America.

Of course, the elements I've just outlined are not true for all who describe themselves using the language of American Evangelicalism, or even for Pentecostalism. The network is too diffused and diverse for a single description to possibly encompass them. Admittedly, my short summary risks generalizing and simplifying in ways that this essay aims to make more complex, namely the networked political theology attendant to Christians in American who practice contemporary Praise and Worship. Nevertheless, it is important to attempt to describe them because it is from within these religious and liturgical contexts that the above-mentioned political positions have emerged and have continued to wield significance in public political and religious discourse.

With this geographic and political context in hand, we return to the question of this essay: why use musical worship events to engage in these political protests? Though Feucht's events follow the well-worn path of urban evangelical proselytizers, something different is happening in Feucht's events from characteristic approaches in American Evangelicalism's past: the worship music itself is the main event, not the "warm-up act" to the headlining preacher. The performance of music does spiritual and political work.

3. Worship Music in the Public Plaza

Liturgical history testifies to a long precedent of worship gatherings outside the doors of the church, from riverside baptisms to stational liturgies, liturgical dramas to public theater and more. Consequently, scholars have begun to consider the role of liturgy in public spaces (such as the urban context) through the broader discourse on "public theology." Foley has suggested that "considering liturgy as an act of public theology presupposed that many, if not most, of those who will interpret the meaning of the worship event will be from outside the faith community." (Foley 2008, p. 31) Therefore, a discussion of meaning (and who constructs it) is central. Likewise, Klomp and Marchand have suggested that because rituals of Christian worship have extended into extra-ecclesial spaces, new modes and methods are required for studying these "sacro-soundscapes" that extend both beyond liturgical studies, ecclesiology, and congregational music studies (Klomp and Barnard 2017). However, such a description has already been provided in part by Ingalls (2018) using the language of "modes of congregating", a framework developed to expand the scope of ecclesiology. Ingalls accounts for public worship gatherings such as Feucht's as one "mode" in this expanded frame of religious musical practices among practitioners of evangelical worship (including charismatics and Pentecostals).

The question of the meaning(s) of Feucht's events has been a challenge in the reception of Feucht's gatherings between and beyond discrete communities of practice (as described in the introduction). It is important to note, however, that given the pervasiveness of Praise and Worship practices across the globe (Ingalls and Yong 2015), more may be understood publicly than is understood in the related academic discourse on public liturgical practices. This study thus employs multiple sources and points of analysis for (re)constructing possible meaning(s) among Pentecostals practicing their religious commitments in the public square. Importantly, my study here diverges from "public theology" proper in that it is an attempt to describe to an academic liturgical studies audience how the practitioners themselves understand the meaning of their practices, not to provide an account of Feucht's events as interpreted by various publics.

Within recent Evangelical, Charismatic, and Pentecostal contexts, public worship music gatherings (or "worship concerts", as some prefer) have become somewhat commonplace at least since Graham Kendrick's Praise March movement in the late 1980s and early 1990s. Though Kendrick is from the U.K., his published books on Praise marches became standard material amongst U.S. Evangelicals. Many will remember the song that takes its name from its iconic chorus by Kendrick: "Shine Jesus Shine." The Praise March Movement took Praise and Worship into the streets in the form of a parade. These marches were an expression both of the Lordship of Christ and a mechanism for spiritual warfare in the city as the practice of Praise and Worship became visible and mainstream (Ingalls 2018, pp. 142–71). Beyond local events, it has become commonplace for worship leaders to wield an increasingly influential level of celebrity within Christian media networks through megachurch platforms and mega-conferences like the annual Passion conference in Atlanta, Georgia or the Hillsong Conference in Sydney, Australia (Busman 2015). These conferences have made worship leaders like Chris Tomlin and David Crowder (Passion) and Darlene Zschech and Joel Houston (Hillsong) household names. These worship music mega-conferences have only grown in significance especially since the early 2000s. Thus worship leaders have played an increasingly important role as public religious figures alongside well-known pastors and other cultural commentators (Ward 2020).

Yet there is something new and distinct happening here with #letusworship. It is more than just the public or urban settings that make Feucht's events noteworthy. Unlike public liturgical practices of the past, why is it that Feucht has chosen worship music in particular as the tool with which he rages against what he perceives to be the politically-motivated repression of Christian worship in America? Though the motivation for his events have stirred up confusion among those who have seen them as a negligent risk to public health at best and willful "superspreader" events at worst (Hudak 2020), his response is intelligible (if still objectionable) when you understand his theology of worship.

4. Feucht's Worship Theology

To understand why worship music is understood as the appropriate response for these Pentecostals to perceived religious oppression requires that I outline a theology of worship that enjoys widespread popularity today. I'll simply call it "Praise and Worship theology" even though it is not monolithic. Ingalls and Yong estimate that nearly one-quarter of the world's Christians practice some form of Praise and Worship (Ingalls and Yong 2015). One very prominent stream of this theology emerged out of the Latter Rain Revival movement of the late 1940s.

The core of this theology is that Praise and Worship manifests God's presence. Liturgical historian Lester Ruth has traced this theology back to a Pentecostal preacher named Reg Layzell in 1946 who popularized the idea that "God inhabits praise", based on Psalm 22:3 (Ruth and Lim 2021). By the late 1970s, a rich and diverse biblical theology had developed around this and other teachings as they became understood through the theological prism of the present-day Restoration of the Tabernacle of David (Perez 2021). Two key verses helped center this scripture. First, Acts 15:16 (quoting Amos 9:11) and the prophecy of the restoration of the Tabernacle of David (read as a restoration of the worship practices associated therein). Second, Hebrews 13:15 on offering a 'sacrifice of praise with our lips,' bringing together the sense that an ongoing sacrifice was still required by God and that the sacrifice was of audible (sung) praise.

Thus, the restoration of the Tabernacle of David centered sung, musical praise as the primary liturgical act restored by King David (see also 1 Chronicles 15). Consequently, in Praise and Worship circles, Praise and Worship practice became synonymous with music-making. Binders of new songs based on the Psalms and Old Testament prophets were written or 'received' by the inspiration of the Holy Spirit. Though music had been a primary feature in Latter Rain worship since the late 1940s, the wave of theological reflection on the Tabernacle of David in the late 1970s and early 1980s led to the emphasis on music as the quintessential expression over and above spoken praise or prayer—two other prominent features associated with early Latter Rain worship practices. As Latter Rain theologians continued to search for scripture's witness on worship, they found that praise's multiple meanings were associated with access to God's power in the life of Israel, a power that could be also be accessed in the present day.[5] The emphasis on music-making continued to move into the mainstream as it coincided with other streams of theological emphasis on music in worship; echoes of Praise and Worship's theological themes can still be heard across a wide range of musical artists and songs.

This theology and worship practice came of age in the late 1970s and 1980s as it was mainstreamed and mixed with other Pentecostal movements like the Word of Faith movement and the Vineyard Church movement (Park et al. 2016). The worship theology of the movement became mainstream in other evangelical, charismatic, and Pentecostal groups through conferences, missionary support networks, and the popularity of Integrity's Hosanna! Music, among other features (Perez 2020). Many of the large churches and church-based worship music groups that are popular today (and/or music labels) have been directly or indirectly influenced by the Latter Rain network and its theologians: Bethel Church (Redding, CA, USA), Gateway Church (Southlake, TX, USA), Hillsong (Sydney, Australia), International House of Prayer (IHOP; Kansas City, MO, USA), and others.

When Feucht says #letusworship, he doesn't mean a simple gathering where Christians pray, read the Bible, and hear a sermon—though that could be part of a larger worship gathering. He means a musical event in particular where Christians sing praises to God. These gatherings are important because Praise and Worship, as the tradition built on Psalm 22:3 teaches, is the normal way Christians encounter God's presence (Snider Andrews 2020). This has become the mainstream assumption of a vast majority of Pentecostals, charismatics, and evangelicals worldwide (Ingalls and Yong 2015; Ruth and Lim 2021).

5. Worshiping at the Seat of Power

If, for Pentecostals, Praise and Worship is about accessing or encountering God's presence, it is also about accessing God's power. When God is present, God acts powerfully and responds to our prayers. Psalm 22:3 is seen as a promise, read as: 'if you praise me, I will come.' Many Pentecostal preachers, teachers, and theologians over the years have highlighted this theme. The sense of God's powerful presence is also magnified through one of the dominant images invoked in Praise and Worship: an enthroned, Kingly God. That is, God has (or should have) political power above all.

Consider this historical example of a representative teaching by Barry Griffing, a Pentecostal pastor and conference leader at the International Worship Symposium. The Symposium was the largest annual worship-focused conference in the U.S. of its era and functioned as a key node in disseminating teachings on Praise and Worship throughout the broader network of Pentecostal, charismatic, and evangelical Christians. At the 1982 conference in Detroit, Michigan, Griffing taught that when ancient Israel restored the practice of Praise and Worship as modeled in David's tabernacle, the nation experienced "spiritual, moral, and military blessing." The direct implication here was that if we too restore Praise and Worship here in the United States in the present day, we can receive those same national blessings today. Of course, Washington D.C. is both an urban space and the political center of the U.S. Indeed, the Symposium took the conference to Constitution Hall and the Washington Mall in 1986 (and saw the highest numbers of attendees) to seek God's national blessings through their Praise and Worship (Perez 2021, pp. 123–30).

In the present day, when Feucht brought his events to places like the steps of the courthouse in Nashville (after a local ordinance banned some types of public gatherings) and culminated the series of events on the Washington Mall in Washington D.C., he was foregrounding this sense of accessing God's presence and power to change the political climate. Indeed, the prominent Pentecostal preacher at Feucht's event on the Washington Mall (25 October 2020), Jentezen Franklin, invoked a theology of praise to rationalize the potential power of the event. Beginning his sermon by telling the gathered crowd, "I don't know if you understand how powerful what we're doing is right now." Franklin invoked the Tabernacle (of David) using Job 36 and the text's use of the water cycle as a metaphor.

> If you want to know what the noise of the Tabernacle, or Praise and Worship, is all about, you have to understand [that] it's about rain. No worship? No rain. Little worship? Little Rain. Rain represents the Holy Spirit. Rain represents righteousness. Rain presents revival. Rain represents miracles, signs, and wonders. Rain is what we need in America and in this world. There are nine expressions in worship the Bible that are invisible vapors that create clouds. Three of them are done with your mouth. You don't just think about it and love him in your heart, but you're supposed to open your mouth and vocalize, verbalize. (Feucht 2020)

Though he emphasized the verbal expressions at greater length, Franklin went on to lead the crowd in short acts encompassing all nine of the verbal and bodily expressions of praise he alluded to. The object of offering God these praises, Franklin told the crowd, was to cause a precipitation God's presence and blessings. Their acts of praise are like water vapors going up into the heavens until "the cloud gets thick and the rain falls."

Accessing God's power in this way is important for doing spiritual work in both individuals and communities. Franklin begins the setup to his closing saying that "demons can't swim" and that the "devil likes dry places." At the climax of his short sermon, Franklin powerfully exhorts the cheering crowd, "American needs a washing! American needs a river! American needs rain! So send up the worship! Send up the praise. Send up the shouts and give him glory!" By coming to the Capitol for this worship music event, Franklin is suggesting that worshippers are preparing for the release of God's power that focuses on the symbolic center of power at the U.S. capitol and extends across the U.S.[6] A very similar message is encoded in Feucht's song "When We Praise" performed at the same event. The song's chorus says, "When we praise/every stronghold breaks/prison doors will shake/the gates of Hell will not prevail."

For Pentecostals, the impulse to go to the halls of power and invoke change has enjoyed renewed theological attention through a concept called the "Seven Mountain Mandate." This scripturally-derived mandate organizes culture and society—including government—into seven areas over which Christians are intended to exercise dominion and establish the Kingdom of God on earth. As a primary liturgical act and spiritual tool, Praise and Worship has become a concrete avenue for pursuing the fulfillment of this mandate. A prominent book within Pentecostal circles on the subject and details of this theology of dominion has been co-written by Bethel Church pastor Bill Johnson and Lance Wallnau (conservative media personality and author) (Wallnau and Johnson 2013). Thus, Praise and Worship does more than build in-group cohesion around political issues among worshippers but is understood to have concrete power to exercise dominion over government and ultimately overturning the laws and policies like the mask mandates that prevent Christian religious expression (read: congregational singing)—legislation that can only be attributed to evil forces and people at the level of state and federal government.

Feucht's #letusworship campaign itinerary planned to culminate at the 25 October 2020 event in Washington, D.C. described above, though he has continued to host events since then (Jenkins 2020). This is not just a show of political power like any other demonstration in Washington D.C., it also has spiritual—even "end-times"—significance as they believe Praise and Worship releases God's power in the spiritual, physical, and political realms. It is why Feucht, as with many Pentecostal revivalists, reports healings and conversions as signs of God's presence in his events and relies on these as the Holy Spirit's validation of his whole movement. In both Franklin's preaching and Feucht's music the legacy of a theology built on Psalm 22:3 remains clear as the link between sung praise and God's powerful presence is direct and consequential means for accomplishing political ends.

6. Worshiping at the Site of Conflict

While Feucht highlights that his worship gatherings are primarily protests against restrictions on church gatherings, his rallies have been also held in places like Portland, OR, Minneapolis, MN, and Kenosha, WI—sites of prominent BLM protests that often turned into showdowns with police. These urban settings are important to Feucht because they reveal a spiritual disturbance at work prompting the protests (not to mention the greater saturation of media attention already focused there). As above, the urban context of Feucht's events are important contexts for the implicit and explicit work that Praise and Worship is meant to accomplish. Notably, Feucht's early description of his worship protests used the tag line, "riots to revivals." The tagline here suggests that "riots" (an overt escalation of the word "protests") themselves are spiritually depraved sites in need of a "revival." Thus, Feucht's gatherings gain a double-valence concerning who the spiritual enemies are: both (the spiritual forces behind) governmental leaders who would place restrictions on church gatherings and those protesting racism and police brutality.

For Feucht, Praise and Worship is the weapon for defeating those spiritual/political enemies just as it was for ancient Israel. Turning again to the archives of Praise and Worship theological teachings, this perspective has been referred to as "The Jehoshaphat Principle" (Griffing 1989). That is, just as in the case with King Jehoshaphat, the worshippers (read: musicians) go out ahead of the army to secure its spiritual victory by bringing about God's presence through praise. More than just urban contexts in general as sites for waging spiritual combat, the particular locations are significant. Powers and principalities (such as those referenced in the Jentezen Franklin sermon above) are understood to be associated with particular geographic locations, a teaching known as "spiritual mapping." C. Peter Wagner has been a loud voice in articulating this now-common Pentecostal theology of place through his writing in books like *Breaking Strongholds in Your City: How to Use Spiritual Mapping to Make Your Prayers More Strategic, Effective, and Targeted*, one volume in a series dedicated to prayer and spiritual warfare (Wagner 1993). This rationale brings to the forefront the theological importance for Feucht to go to the places where prominent protests (and potentially strong demonic activities) are happening. In using Praise and Worship as spiritual warfare, the songs of Feucht's gatherings are anthemic and the overall tone is joyful and unrelentingly positive in the belief that the worship changes the emotional atmosphere as it changes the spiritual and political situation (Payne 2021).

Because God's spiritual power is released through musical worship in general, song choice is quite powerful. Songs like Feucht's "When We Praise" (quoted above) are relatively forward in describing their political connections, as are other songs used at his gatherings. Martin Smith's "Did you Feel the Mountains Tremble" and the line in its the chorus "Open up the doors and let the music play" and Feucht's other song "Let Everything (Praise the Lord)" both clearly identify the desired ends in their lyrics. Other sources have been coopted into Feucht's service as well. One popular anthem being sung at Feucht's and other recent gatherings (Boorstein and Bailey 2020) is "Great Are You Lord", a song by the group All Sons and Daughters. In the worship protest context, the line from the chorus, "It's your breath in our lungs, so we pour out your praise" becomes a clear and defiant cry against governmental restrictions on congregational singing and mask requirements while it also signals a veiled reference to George Floyd's famous "I can't breathe" statement.

7. Concluding Remarks

Feucht is just one node in a long line of Christians engaged in public political demonstrations in urban contexts. Though the tactics of his response to pandemic restrictions appear novel, they build on a theological and musical tradition going back many decades. It is important to note, too, that this theology of Praise and Worship is not simply a "white evangelical" practice. His tactics and ends may be unique, but shared theologies of worship are operationalized in Black Churches and Latinx Churches. See, for example, the work of early Praise and Worship pioneers like Judith McAllister and her album "Send Judah First" or Marcos Witt's song "Sana Nuestra Tierra" ("Heal Our Land"), popular throughout Latin America. Therefore, we can say that this Pentecostal, musicalized theology of worship has become entangled in white Christian Nationalist discourses around religious freedom for Feucht in ways that are not entirely due to their common root of worship theology.

Looking into the backdrop of Feucht's worship theology provides another lens for making sense of the present pandemic and the weaving together of liturgical-theological and political commitments. Together with other analyses, we can gain a clearer sense of how history, the politics of pandemic response, social unrest, and theology have come together in novel ways to form liturgical practices. What is at stake in addressing the problem of the pandemic is more than political and ideological differences but complex and deeply rooted theological commitments that have long been practiced in worshipping communities and forming Christian identities. It would be dangerous to undervalue either the liturgical-theological nature of what is at stake for these Pentecostals or how Christian worshippers are wielding theology to powerfully shape the way justice and social action are imagined and enacted.

Funding: This research received no external funding.

Institutional Review Board Statement: Not applicable.

Informed Consent Statement: Not applicable.

Data Availability Statement: Not applicable.

Conflicts of Interest: The author declares no conflict of interest.

Notes

1 Perhaps the most scandalous was a t-shirt design created in response to a headline about Feucht's events by Rolling Stone Magazine, suggesting that that his events were potentially COVID-19 "superspreader" events. The t-shirts read "Jesus Christ: Super-Spreader." See "Well, Sean Feucht Is Now Selling 'Jesus Christ: Super-Spreader' T-Shirts, Apparently" *Relevant Magazine* (20 November 2020) https://www.relevantmagazine.com/current/well-sean-feucht-is-now-selling-jesus-christ-super-spreader-t-shirts-apparently/ (accessed 23 November 2021).

2 In this essay, I treat Pentecostals as a subset of evangelicals in the broadest sense. Following Monique Ingalls, I suggest that there is a shared social imaginary between within and between evangelicals, Pentecostals, and charismatics that is constituted by worship music and its various "modes of congregating" (Ingalls 2018).

3 In positioning his protests against Gov. Newsom's policies, Feucht is hardly unique. See also Sam Kestenbaum's reporting in The Washington Post on other evangelical churches in California that have positioned their worship service policies in direct opposition to Gov. Newsom (Kestenbaum 2021).

4 For descriptions of some of these events see Mayfield 2020 on Feucht's event in Portland, Spera 2020 on the Mayor of New Orleans publicly condemning Feucht's event there, and Duin 2020 on Feucht sidestepping a ban on his concert by calling it a "protest."

5 In particular, the interpretation of the seven primary Hebrew words that have been translated into English as "praise" in (Ottaway Forthcoming)

6 This isn't the only time Feucht has partnered with Franklin. In a different video of a sermon preached at Franklin's church when they hosted Feucht in October of 2021 Franklin praises Feucht and his team for "going all over the nation and some of the most troubled cities in America and declaring the name of Jesus." His sermon opens by making a direct connection between worship, God's presence, and receiving healing and help. See "Let Us Worship | Jentezen Franklin" https://www.youtube.com/watch?v=AC5N88IDvGQ (accessed 23 November 2021).

References

Baldovin, John F. 1987. *The Urban Character of Christian Worship: The Origins, Development, and Meaning of Stational Liturgy*. Orientalia Christiana Analecta; 228. Rome: Pont. Institutum Studiorum Orientalium.

Boorstein, Michelle, and Sarah Pulliam Bailey. 2020. Prayer March Draws Thousands to the Mall Seeking Healing for the Nation. *Washington Post*. September 26. Available online: https://www.washingtonpost.com/local/social-issues/prayer-march-national-mall/2020/09/26/e401f184-002f-11eb-b555-4d71a9254f4b_story.html (accessed on 29 November 2021).

Busman, Joshua Kalin. 2015. (Re)Sounding Passion: Listening to American Evangelical Worship Music, 1997–2015. Ph.D. thesis, The University of North Carolina, Chapel Hill, NC, USA.

Du Mez, Kristin Kobes. 2020. *Jesus and John Wayne: How White Evangelicals Corrupted a Faith and Fractured a Nation*, 1st ed. New York: W.W. Norton & Company, Inc.

Duin, Julia. 2020. Christian Musician Sean Feucht Held Defiant Seattle Worship Protest After Concert Was Banned. *Religion News Service*. September 8 sec. Arts & Culture. Available online: https://religionnews.com/2020/09/08/christian-musician-sean-feucht-seattle-bethel-worship-protest-concert-covid-19/ (accessed on 10 November 2021).

Feucht, Sean. 2020. The Noise of His Tabernacle—Sean Feucht—Pastor Jentezen Franklin—Let Us Worship—DC. Available online: https://www.youtube.com/watch?v=270b05R4nPI&feature=youtu.be&ab_channel=SeanFeucht (accessed on 8 November 2021).

Foley, Edward. 2008. Engaging the Liturgy of the World: Worship as Public Theology. *Studia Liturgica* 38: 31–52. [CrossRef]

Griffing, Steve. 1989. The Jehoshaphat Principle. In *An Anthology of Articles on Restoring Praise & Worship to the Church*. Edited by David Blomgren, Douglas Christoffel and Dean Smith. Shippensburg: Revival Press.

Hudak, Joseph. 2020. Jesus Christ, Superspreader? *Rolling Stone*, October 12. Available online: https://www.rollingstone.com/culture/culture-news/sean-feucht-preacher-covid-1074213/ (accessed on 8 November 2021).

Ingalls, Monique Marie, and Amos Yong, eds. 2015. *The Spirit of Praise: Music and Worship in Global Pentecostal-Charismatic Christianity*. University Park: The Pennsylvania State University Press.

Ingalls, Monique Marie. 2018. *Singing the Congregation: How Contemporary Worship Music Forms Evangelical Community*. Oxford: Oxford University Press.

Jenkins, Jack. 2020. Sean Feucht's 'Finale' Worship Protest on the National Mall Included More Politics than Usual. *Religion News Service (blog)*, October 26. Available online: https://religionnews.com/2020/10/26/sean-feuchts-finale-worship-protest-on-the-national-mall-included-more-politics-than-usual/ (accessed on 12 November 2021).

Kestenbaum, Sam. 2021. Since This California Church Began Flouting Pandemic Restrictions, Attendance Has Surged. *The Washington Post*, February 26. Available online: https://www.washingtonpost.com/religion/2021/02/26/godspeak-calvary-covid-rob-mccoy/ (accessed on 29 November 2021).

Klomp, Mirella, and Marcel Barnard. 2017. Sacro-Soundscapes: Interpreting Contemporary Ritual Performances of Sacred Music through the Case of The Passion in the Netherlands. *International Journal of Practical Theology* 21: 240–58. [CrossRef]

"Let Us Worship." n.d. Available online: https://www.letusworship.us/ (accessed on 29 November 2021).

Mayfield, D. L. 2020. How a Sean Feucht Worship Service Convinced Me I Am No Longer an Evangelical. *Religion News Service*. September 23 sec. Opinion. Available online: https://religionnews.com/2020/09/23/how-a-sean-feucht-worship-service-convinced-me-i-am-no-longer-an-evangelical/ (accessed on 29 November 2021).

Mulder, Mark T. 2015. *Shades of White Flight: Evangelical Congregations and Urban Departure*. New Brunswick: Rutgers University Press.

Omri, Elisha. 2010. Taking the (Inner) City of God: Ambiguities of Urban Social Engagement among Conservative White Evangelicals. In *The Fundamentalist City? Religiosity and the Remaking of Urban Space*. Edited by Nezar AlSayyad and Mejgan Massoumi. London: Taylor & Francis, pp. 235–56.

Ottaway, Jonathan. Forthcoming. The Seven Hebrew Words for Praise: Pentecostal Interpretations of Scripture in Liturgical Theology. *Worship*. (forthcoming 2022).

Park, Andy, Lester Ruth, and Cindy Rethmeier. 2016. *Worshiping with the Anaheim Vineyard: The Emergence of Contemporary Worship*. Grand Rapids: Eerdmans.

Payne, Leah. 2021. The Trump Shall Sound: Politics, Pentecostals, and the Shofar at the Capitol Riots. *Political Theology Network*, September 2. Available online: https://politicaltheology.com/the-trump-shall-sound-politics-pentecostals-and-the-shofar-at-the-capitol-riots/ (accessed on 27 September 2021).

Perez, Adam. 2020. Enthroned Upon Praise: The Early History and Theology of Integrity's Hosanna! Music. In *Essays on the History of Contemporary Praise and Worship*. Eugene: Pickwick Press.

Perez, Adam A. 2021. "All Hail King Jesus": The International Worship Symposium and the Making of Praise and Worship History, 1977–1989. Th.D. dissertation, Duke University Divinity School, Duke, NC, USA.

Ruth, Lester, and Swee Hong Lim. 2021. *A History of Contemporary Praise and Worship: Understanding the Ideas That Reshaped the Protestant Church*. Grand Rapids: Baker Academic.

Snider Andrews, Emily. 2020. *Exploring Evangelical Sacramentality: Modern Worship Music and the Possibility of Divine-Human Encounter*. Ph.D. dissertationPasadena: Fuller Theological Seminary.

Spera, Keith. 2020. Sean Feucht, Lauren Daigle Preached Irresponsibility at French Quarter Worship Event. *NOLA.Com*, November 10. Available online: https://www.nola.com/entertainment_life/keith_spera/article_44b2ea74-2380-11eb-b0e3-87e81927bff8.html (accessed on 29 November 2020).

Wagner, C. Peter. 1993. *Breaking Strongholds in Your City: How to Use Spiritual Mapping to Make Your Prayers More Strategic, Effective, and Targeted*. Ventura: Regal Books.

Wallnau, Lance, and Bill Johnson. 2013. *Invading Babylon: The 7 Mountain Mandate*. Shippensburg: Destiny Image.

Ward, Pete. 2020. *Celebrity Worship*. New York: Routledge.

religions

MDPI

Article

Venezuelan Evangelical Digital Diaspora, Pandemics, and the Connective Power of Contemporary Worship Music

Fernando Adolfo Mora [1,*] and Enrique García Martínez [2]

1 Bioengineering and Applied Biophysics Group, Simón Bolívar University, Caracas 89000, Venezuela
2 Entrecristianos, 28051 Madrid, Spain; ejgarciam@gmail.com
* Correspondence: famorac@gmail.com

Abstract: During 2020–2021, the COVID-19 pandemics exacerbated the use of digital communication tools for the general population as well as for migrant and diasporic communities. Due to social distancing requirements, church activities had to be suspended or restricted, therefore, local congregations and denominations had to incorporate social media as part of their regular worship channels in an unprecedented way. At the same time, these new spaces opened an opportunity for diasporas to reconnect with their churches back home, and to participate in digital worship projects. In this paper, we study the case of the digital worship collective *Adorando en Casa* (AeC), which was started at the onset of the pandemics, producing several crowdsourced original musical compositions, uploaded in popular social media sites, and distributed via messaging apps. We focus on the reasons for participation of Venezuelan musicians and singers from different regions in the country, and from the large diaspora of Venezuelan Evangelicals. Additionally, we analyze the characteristics, structure, and theology of some of the songs recorded, to show how the concept of a digital diasporic spiritual consciousness is powerfully expressed through worship music.

Keywords: pandemics; contemporary worship; digital worship; COVID-19; coronamusic; digital diasporas; migration

1. The Rise of Digital Religion during the Pandemics

Since early 2020, the COVID-19 pandemic has created all kinds of crises in contemporary society. Its effects on individuals, families, groups, organizations, and nations are yet to be known and understood. As Deborah Lupton and Karen Willis put it, "the COVID crisis is a complex and ever-thickening entanglement of people with other living things, place, space, objects, time, discourse and culture" (Lupton and Willis 2021). It has trespassed its physical health dimensions, as a viral disease that produces an inflammatory response that affects different body systems, with life-threatening cardio-respiratory complications, to become a relational disease that has disrupted all spheres of society. Christianity worldwide was thoroughly affected by the COVID-19 pandemic. All over the world, churches were asked to put regular services on hold. Unexpectedly, the digitalization of rituals, Bible studies, discipleship groups, church services, counselling, as well as the transmission of religious knowledge and information, and the like, went from being just an idea of some religious entrepreneurs, to becoming an urgent need. Due to the lack of experience, many churches started to replicate with great difficulty in the digital space what was commonly done face–face. Basically, we were witnessing the accelerated rebooting of offline activities to a whole different space with a set of powerful media affordances designed for patterns of interaction, information flow, knowledge dissemination, and wisdom elicitation, that were completely novel and, in some cases, somewhat incompatible, with a face–face Christian culture.

Previous researchers had envisioned a progressive incorporation of digital technologies in religious practices, adopting the term *digital religion* to describe the intersection between religious traditions and the evolving and ubiquitous digital technologies (Campbell and Evolvi 2020). Nevertheless, the COVID-19 pandemic represented an abrupt change to the practice of religion all over the world. The different ways that churches and Christians in general responded to these challenges implied the introduction of new tools, new practices, the adaptation of existing platforms, and a greater dependency on digital media, and information and telecommunication technology in their everyday lives during the lockdowns. Without intending it, Christianity arrived at a point where digital religion practices became essential to any believer, in different church traditions, and all over the world. It was possible to consider in a tangible, and somewhat massive way, how social networks, telecommunication technology, data management, new media, and the like, were being incorporated by believers "into their everyday life and into their patterns of worship and religiosity" (Campbell and Evolvi 2020). It was not simply a matter of what new platform, software, or gadget could be used, but how its use was shaped by the spirituality and theological views of the potential users. Thus, this real-life situation forced researchers to pay close attention to "existential, ethical, and political aspects of digital religion, as well as issues of gender, race, class, ethnicity, sexuality." (p. 7). In a way, the practice of religion during the pandemic became an immense laboratory where many different initiatives were started, some successful and lasting, others less effective, and many others with purposes that were charged with conspirative theories and political messages.

Some years before the pandemic, Helland stated that digital religion goes beyond the packaging of liturgies into new digital media; instead, it involves a careful conceptualization of the "societal and cultural components we associate with religion with the elements we associate with a digital society" (Helland 2016). Taking this into account, there are some aspects that conditioned the reengineering of church services in digital spaces during the COVID-19 crisis, such as the individualism and commodification introduced by the widespread use of the Internet; the accessibility to huge amounts of content and knowledge that produces a weakening of religious authority; the networked nature of digital media which leads to the flattening of religious structures, their decentralization, and deterritorialization; and also the immediacy and ubiquity of networks and social media that induce changes in the temporal logic of users, and modify the levels of commitment to communities. To classify the attempts to create digital spaces during the pandemic, the framework proposed by Piotr Siuda, that combines two contrasting axes, *information* vs. *participation*, and *innovation* vs. *tradition*, is useful (Siuda 2021). According to that, the first axis informs about the level of participation and creativity of the implementations, which implies also a more varied and intense use of digital technologies. The second axis informs about how churches or organizations deploy their existing power dynamics, if the level of information is controlled, and if the communication protocol follows rigid patterns or is more spontaneous. Siuda (2021) also proposes several questions which serve to map any digital religion initiative within the proposed two-axes framework, that can be used to investigate our case study, such as: which digital tools are used? What kind of spiritual activities are facilitated? How about the characteristics of the religious experiences in the digital space? Additionally, how these digital religion practices are incorporated within the existing church structures or if they occur as independent initiatives?

As we will see in the following sections, our case study is not just an implementation done by some tech savvy Christian entrepreneurs, but by a group of believers that, as Sheldon and Campbell (2021) state, "have rejected the dualism of technology as distinct from the spiritual" realm, understanding their use of technology as a vehicle for God's manifestation, in a world troubled by COVID-19 and other difficult situations such as political persecution and migration. For this reason, we find that the framework proposed by Heidi Campbell (Campbell 2005) is useful to analyze the ways that the users in our case study view their approach to digital tools, and how they describe God's presence or work in their technology mediated implementations. In this framework, any religious digital space can be seen from four different perspectives: (1) As a *spiritual network*, where people connect in virtual spaces and find meaningful spiritual experiences together; (2) As a *sacramental space* where God can visit and communicate with the believers, which implies that certain forms of spiritual experiences can be facilitated digitally, and where a sense of holiness can be found; (3) As *a tool* for evangelism, when it is used for missional purposes, or, as a vehicle for the dissemination of religious ideas, when it serves to communicate certain theologies or practices among different religious communities; and, (4) As *a place* where the practice of religion involve the use of technologies for the daily practice of faith, and for the digital interconnection with other believers through virtual communities of faith. In the final section of this paper, we will revisit this framework in the context of our case study.

2. COVID-19 Pandemics and Digital Worship

Although streaming church services was not new, it was reserved to certain churches such as those employing a multisite model, where both online and offline audiences participated in the same church service (Campbell and De Lashmutt 2014). However, the COVID-19 pandemic forced almost all local churches, regardless of their size, to find solutions to allow their members to continue worshiping together and connecting as a fellowship, despite the severe lockdowns that were imposed in many regions in the world.

One quick fix to the problem of church attendance during lockdowns was to launch Zoom-based services. The Zoom user base had been growing for several years among educational institutions, because, in some ways, its design mimics a traditional classroom. During the pandemic, church online meetings using Zoom became very popular because the power dynamics of classical attractional churches change very little. In the case of Pentecostal/Charismatic congregations, which rely so much on contemporary worship music expressions, where voices and bodies play a major part of the liturgic experience, a Zoom meeting may seem awkward and incomplete. Worship music has gained a central role as part of the liturgy that was developed after the Jesus Movement in the 1960s and 1970s, due to the use of rock/pop contemporary music styles, dance, congregational participation in spontaneous singing, prophecy, or prayer, which, for the most part, had acquired a performative concert like characteristic. In Pentecostal/Charismatic (P/C) contemporary worship models, sacramentality plays a fundamental role in their theology (Lim and Ruth 2017). Based on Old Testament passages about the enactment of David's Tabernacle (Pérez 2021), a new liturgy emerged, based on the expectation that, if it was well planned and executed, God would be present during the praises of the gathered people. This type of worship experience currently dominates most of the liturgical models employed in Latin America, in what has been termed as the *Pentecostalization* of the Evangelical church in the region (Gladwin 2015).

In contemporary P/C worship, there is a "desire to *encounter the divine* through music, and a sense that, when God is present, He is present in active power" (Lim and Ruth 2017, pp. 130–31). In the sacramental theology of P/C contemporary praise and worship, "the worshiper is lifted up into heaven, into God's presence, into the throne room in which God resides" (Snider Andrews 2019). Intimacy with God is achieved through music that expresses love to God, such that the believer can experience God's presence as real and overwhelming. It seems, at first, that social media and digital worship spaces are incompatible with these experiences of the presence of God. At first glance, the technological affordances available in the existing social media applications are very limited to allow for remote worship in such a way that, praise and worship flow can be facilitated in a seamless way, and to allow the collective display of the type of emotional expressions that a worship service entails (Addo 2021).

Since the beginning of the pandemic music listening, music crafting, and singing seemed like a natural way to withstand the lockdowns. Some authors have started to look at the variety of "practices of listening to, playing, dancing to, composing, rehearsing, improvising, discussing, exploring, and innovating musical products" (Hansen et al. 2021), under the newly coined term of *coronamusic* to designate musical expressions originated during the COVID-19 pandemic. Since a typology of coronamusic has not been proposed yet, it might be possible to call the *musicking* (Small 1999), that is, all the sonic and social relationships that are part of worship music making, listening, participating, interacting, experiencing, dancing, video making, that happened during the pandemic, *coronaworship*.

Music video streaming has been positively associated with the severity of COVID-19 lockdown policies, and with the increased time spent at home (Sim et al. 2020). Youtube can be both, a source of emotion and a meeting point for certain communities (Rosenbusch et al. 2019). In the case of worship music, the richness of the images, the abundance of emotional display, the feeling of the music, are all factors that could produce an authentic online worship experience. Compared to worship leaders in church settings, worship music videos creators on Youtube are subject to a large range of responses from channel subscribers and casual visitors. Authenticity in the worship performance is perceived by followers from the actual way the video is produced, which is typically more grass-root, semi-professional, quite different than highly produced, well written scripts, professionally acted, video clips. In other words, "authenticity [is] established in ... a dialogic relationship" between creators and viewers as part of the conventions of the social media platform in use (Cunningham and Craig 2017). Under these premises, it is possible to assume that *Worship Music Video* (WMV) streaming exploded during the COVID-19 crisis. Prior to the pandemic, Monique Ingalls had studied different kinds of Youtube worship music videos, focusing her study on user-generated WMVs combining "song lyrics, scriptural texts, and images to commercial recordings of worship songs", which, according to her, is the most popular way of accessing worship music on the web (Ingalls 2016).

Although WMV's help to fill the gap left by the impossibility of face-face gatherings, the element of mutual listening, collaborative musicking, and congregational singing is difficult to emulate just by watching Youtube videos. The need to join others to produce a musical creative synergy does not seem to be new in public health crises. According to Chiu, music fulfils the dual role of mood regulation, meditation, emotional healing, and of fostering social cohesion, bonding, connection, and solidarity, in times of isolation (Chiu 2020). For Christians during the lockdowns this meant finding ways to care for each other, to provide for their spiritual and material needs, and to intercede in prayer for the healing of their neighbors, cities, nations, or the world at large. Chiu also relates balcony singing, flash mobs, online musical ensembles, playlist creation, and many other initiatives that were spontaneously put together during the lockdowns around the world, with the singing and music making in other pandemics, such as the Milan plague in 1576. At that time, the singing and recitation of litanies were taken home by order of the city bishop. The singing of praises to God, along with the intercession for those suffering from the plague, continued non-stop, day and night, creating an overwhelming soundscape, which for those in the city reminded of "the roar of rushing waters" in the book of Revelations.

The performative aspect of worship music and the expectation of God's visitation during the stages of call, praise, intimacy, and thanksgiving, which are part of the contemporary P/C music during the liturgical experience, have been very difficult to reproduce in online musicking during the COVID-19 pandemic. This is due, in part, to the technological limitations that networks and software have for joint music making in real time, and to achieve the presence and togetherness that are essential in the worship experience (Onderdijk et al. 2021). With the idea that sound can facilitate the divine encounter, despite the limitations, some events were promoted to do spontaneous improvisations of music over Zoom (Roberts 2021).

Alternative asynchronous ways for cooperative remote musicking were also explored, such as crowdsourcing individual parts that were edited later to produce WMVs published on social media platforms. One well-known example of online coronaworship musicking during COVID-19 lockdowns was the singing of the benediction in Numbers 6:24–26 based on the musical arrangements of Kari Jobe, Cody Carnes, and members from *Elevation Worship* in Charlotte (North Caroline). A crowdsourced version with the contribution of 30 churches was produced under the initiative of a Pittsburgh church, followed by a *UK Blessing* version with 65 churches participating. After that, more than 100 versions from different regions of the world[1], and a global choir live performance coordinated by Elevation Church in May 2020, followed (Fowler 2020). A similar project was the *Irish Blessing*, dedicating the 1000-year-old Irish hymn, *Be Thou my Vision*, to their local health facilities, overburdened with the rapid spread of the SARS-COV-2 virus. The WMV was edited from 500 online submissions, representing over 300 churches in the final crowdsourced video version (McGarry 2020). The resulting WMVs in YouTube of many of these different blessings became viral and, in a way, marked a trend in what coronaworship musicking would look like during the long lockdowns in 2020 and 2021.

Another resource that exploded during the COVID-19 pandemic was the use of WhatsApp religious groups. A 2019 report of 11 emergent economies (PRC 2019) showed that, on average, over 65% of Latin Americans were regular users of WhatsApp, with some countries with more than 72% of penetration (Meher 2022). WhatsApp uses only the cell phone number as identity; thus, the whole contact list automatically becomes a social network. One of the reasons for the fast growth of WhatsApp has to do with the *scalability* of its group feature, because each user can create a group and invite any contact that is in the smartphone, and those invited can repeat the process, thus producing a multiplicative effect. Additionally, there is the possibility of infinite content sharing, defined as *replicability*, some sort of chain effect, where messages are forwarded from user to user, or from group to group, sometimes received by one user repeated times, regardless of its origin or veracity (Pang and Woo 2020).

3. Faith on the Move: Venezuelan Evangelical Digital Diasporas and Worship Music

Venezuelan diaspora has been relentless since the year 2012. Starting in 2015 (Chaves-Gonzalez and Echeverria-Estrada 2020), several waves of Venezuelan migrants have been described in the literature, with a fast and steady growth since 2017. In September of 2021, the United Nations accounted more than 5.7 million Venezuelans that have moved out of the country due to the difficult living conditions, 80% of them were in other Latin American and Caribbean countries (R4V: Plataforma Regional de Coordinación Interagencial 2021). This number of migrants represents around 20% of the country's population according to its most recent national census (Instituto Nacional de Estadística de Venezuela 2011).

In the literature, the term *diaspora* has been employed to describe a large national, cultural, or religious group living in foreign lands (Baumann 2010), dispersed from its homeland due to war, economic, political, ethnic, or religious reasons (Butler 2001). Four basic features characterize a diaspora: (1) The scattering into several destinations, which in the case of Venezuelans, includes almost all Latin American and Caribbean countries, the US, and European nations, with Spain as the main destination; (2) some kind of relationship to homeland has to be present, for example through remittances, or, as we will see below, through different forms of social, cultural, religious and political participation using digital affordances, which can be classified as *social remittances* (Levitt 2007); (3) a consciousness and identity as a group that binds them together and also connects them with the homeland, which is continuously reinforced through messaging groups, associations of migrants, and online activism, or as Vásquez puts it, diasporas: "relate to the homeland through desire, through the unfulfilled longing for a paradise lost and the utopian dreams of a future return to mythic origins" (Vásquez 2008); and also, (4) that the state of dispersion persists long enough such that it cannot be considered only a temporary exile; in this regard, the majority of Venezuelan migrants left the country since 2015, but the conditions for possible return are harder, as political conflict endures.

The religious dimension is another element that binds the diasporic community, and which modulates its relationship with the homeland, and its idealization according to a specific spiritual imagination or worldview. According to a Pew Research Center study, the percentage of *Evangélicos*[2] in Venezuela was growing at about 1% per year, which would lead to more than 20% in 2021 (PRC 2014). Following this pattern, it is safe to say that around 20% of the total Venezuelan diaspora are Evangelicals (García Ayala 2019), without counting those converted in their pilgrimage through countries where evangelical churches are growing quite fast (Pérez Guadalupe 2020). The unique role that digital religion plays here is that these diasporic communities can connect and relate through networks that span through the different host countries where there are Venezuelan migrants. Not only these networks have different topologies, but digital technologies also allow for the creation of many different networks of networks. However, their power rest in the fact that besides the purely relational aspect, the networks of believers also contain multiple "phenomenological realities consisting of narratives, practices, cognitive maps, and microhistories" (Vásquez 2008). This leads us to consider how evangelical migrants incorporate religious networks in the way they live their religion in the diaspora. Thus, documenting diasporic religious network formation during the COVID-19 pandemic in terms of accessibility, type of actors, religious power of members, ways of exchange and communication, digital media employed, type of content shared, formalization, and other aspects, is an important contribution to the understanding of "how religious networks come to be constituted and rooted in a particular space and time and how different kinds of ties come together to form transnational social fields" (Vásquez 2008).

Venezuelan migration waves have occurred during the proliferation of the use of social media and smartphones. Due to the magnitude of social networking usage, researchers have been able to estimate the number of Venezuelan migrants in South America using Facebook (Santos 2018), or to track the flow and routes of migration using Twitter data (Mazzoli et al. 2020). Venezuelan Evangelicals in foreign lands have become true digital diasporic communities (Ponzanesi 2020), recreating identities, sharing opportunities, spreading culture and ideas, and even influencing churches, organizations, and even governments (Alonso and Oiarzabal 2010). The immediacy, fluidity, and frequency of new telecommunication modes facilitates building up trust, intimacy, virtual presence, and the transmission of emotion, which are fundamental for the creation of meaningful religious spaces, especially in Pentecostal and Charismatic expressions of worship and prayer.

When looking at music making by diasporic communities, it is enlightening to consider what Walter Brueggemann has called the *disciplines of readiness* (Brueggemann 1997). By drawing from the experience of the Babylonian exile in the Old Testament, Brueggemann sees the Jews learning to practice such disciplines through dangerous *memories*, dangerous *criticism*, dangerous *promises*, dangerous *new songs*. These disciplines belong to the realm of the ritual and liturgy of the diasporic worshiping community. One of the most powerful vehicles through which memories, criticism, and promises can travel, and reach other diasporic communities in forced exile, are *dangerous new songs* that speak of their homeland and of the new alternatives that are. Artistic forms such as music, can be valuable ways to communicate the difficulties of migrants and diasporic communities in their pilgrimage, such as discrimination, exclusion, and lack of access to basic rights, the sense of loss of the migrant's natural world, of their first loves, or the most cherished dreams, can be captured in songs (Paniagua-Arguedas 2017)[3].

The use of Christian music by diasporic communities has been studied in reference to migrants from African countries, due to the extraordinary growth of their diasporic Pentecostal churches around the world, especially Nigerian congregations in the UK, where music has played a central role in their expansion (Sabar and Kanari 2006). However, very few studies have been done among Latin American Evangelical diasporic communities. Rocha studied the fascination of immigrants from Brazil who were members of Hillsong church in Sidney (Rocha 2017). Adopting Hillsong music as the proper way to worship God, was one way to capture their imaginations, identifying with something powerful, and, at the same time, detaching from the religiosity and legalism of the Pentecostal churches in their homeland. Deborah Berhó observed in Hispanic churches in the state of Oregon that most of the songs used were in Spanish, and they preferred US-Hispanic or Latin American composers in their repertoire (Berhò 2020). Recent research among Peruvian and Bolivian migrants attending a Pentecostal church in Iquique (Chile), observed that, despite the global sound and familiarity of migrants with the repertoire, *nostalgia* was the main feeling evoked by worship music among the diasporic community (Vélez Caro and

Mansilla 2019). However, the pain produced by loneliness, vulnerability, and economic scarcity that migration brings, can be overcome through the rich symbolic imagery and powerful sonic texture that contemporary worship music possess.

In the case of the Venezuelan diasporic communities, migrants who once were pastors, worship leaders, church planters, home group leaders, now work in the host land as Uber drivers, delivering food, doing domestic service, in all kinds of occupations that can provide enough money to pay food and lodging, even as undertakers of COVID-19 fatalities in Lima (Perú) a job that was rejected by locals (Galdos and Somra 2020). The message of hope that the gospel brings is a way of dealing with the hardships of everyday life. One of the coping mechanisms of migrant Evangelical populations, or for those converted while migrating, is to join a church where a solid network of believers can be found. In this situation, music is a very powerful instrument when, as exiles, the diasporic community is trying to reimagine faith and give sense to what is happening to them. Music unites the diasporic community and serves as a vehicle for its identity formation in the host culture. However, this process was completely disrupted for Venezuelan Evangelical migrants during the 2020–2021 COVID-19 pandemic. Regular gatherings in the local churches in the host country had to be suspended, and diasporic communities became virtual and had to rely on new ways to interact and keep united. In the next section, we explore a case study of a digital worship music digital community composed of members from the Venezuelan Evangelical digital diaspora, as well as Christians in the homeland, that was started spontaneously during the COVID-19 pandemic, where both, nostalgia, and hope, for a better situation in Venezuela dominates the poetry, influences the musical style, and dictates the characteristics of the WMVs produced for use by Venezuelan Evangelical churches.

4. Case Study: *Adorando en Casa* as Virtual Communitas

Simons (2009) has defined a case study as "an in-depth exploration from multiple perspectives of the complexity and uniqueness of a particular project, policy, institution, program or system in 'real life'" (p. 21). In this regard, we centered our research interest on *the case* at hand (Starman 2013), as a unique illustrative example of the interaction between different research areas, such as digital religion, religion and migration, digital diasporic communities, and contemporary worship music, within the context of an ongoing complex situation such as the COVID-19 pandemics. The case study is done both retrospectively, by collecting data from different sources, since the beginning of the digital worship community at the onset of the pandemic, and also, through collective reflection of the members of the group as they continue their collaboration through the 4th or 5th wave of the pandemic. We approached this research without proposing any hypothesis, but with the firm idea that we could learn from the case study and identify new areas that require in depth exploration based on the documentation of a real-life experience such as the one we will describe below.

Adorando en Casa (AeC) is a collective of worship leaders, musicians, singers, and pastors that was formed at the beginning of the COVID-19 pandemic in 2020. To study the development of the group, we have reviewed all their productions that were posted on Youtube, looking at the responses and commentaries to these WMVs. Additionally, we analyzed interviews that were done by Evangelical media, as well as the opinion of pastors and other Christian leaders. As a way to obtain a more objective observation, we also asked a Venezuelan musicologist, worship leader and pastor, Wershin Montiel, who is also part of the diaspora, to listen and comment about the lyrics and musical arrangements of the seven songs, produced by AeC, with more visits in their Youtube channel. We also did participatory observation in the WhatsApp group and Telegram channel of AeC for several months, which allowed us to observe the virtual community and the interactions during the processes of music production, times of prayer, or mutual care.

In order to gather direct observations from those who were part of the network, we conducted a digital focus group with eight members located in Toronto—Canada, San Jose—Costa Rica, Quito—Ecuador, and Merida and Valencia in Venezuela, using a Telegram chat, from 4 October to 24 October 2021. The focus group was carried out with three rounds of questions. The first one was targeted to get to know more about the participants and the reasons why those living abroad had left Venezuela. The second batch of questions sought to find out why they had decided to join AeC, and the benefits of being part of the network. The third round allowed the participants in the focus group to reflect on the musical genre and the lyrics of the songs produced collectively by AeC, as well as to consider the impact of the music among Evangelicals in Venezuela. All participants in the focus group had a Pentecostal background, although some had moved to Neo-Pentecostal or New Apostolic Reformation (NAR) churches recently. Of those in the diaspora due to the Venezuelan crisis, only one was still in the process of integration into the new culture. All joined AeC, either because of the need to connect their faith during the pandemic, looking for an opportunity to serve God, or because of the need for friendship. Among the participants of the focus group, it was agreed that through AeC they managed to connect with Venezuela. Besides that, the growing sisterhood and brotherhood among the members of AeC, wherever they may be, allowed for more personal mutual edification, prayer in difficult times, or spiritual renewal. In general terms, all the participants in the focus group wanted to continue producing music together, and staying interconnected, after the pandemic ends.

During the focus group, the participants recognized Ronald Sifontes, a professional musical producer from Mérida in the Venezuelan Andes, as the inspirational leader who started the network. Ronald was forced to close his music recording studio when his work contracts went suddenly to zero in March 2020. At the beginning of the pandemic, he was reminded of a prophetic word received in 1993 from the Mexican worship leader Marcos Barrientos, realizing that the COVID-19 crisis was one of those times that the prophecy spoke about, and that it was important to step out. Immediately, he started to draw from his personal network those worshipers, psalmists, pastors, and musicians, from several churches in the country, and from the Venezuelan diaspora, inviting them to unite and do something in the musical arena. Very quickly, those invited brought more people to the network, such that by early April 2020 a growing WhatsApp group had already been started, and the name for the community was coined: *Adorando en Casa* (Worshipping at home, AeC).

Initially, three objectives were proposed for the network in a Youtube video, stating that it was a space for the expression of worship using different musical styles with the participation of Venezuelans from all over the world, and from all denominations; to encourage participation not only through music, but by developing devotionals, scripture reading, and prayer rooms; and, the composition of new worship songs that reflected the times and the difficulties confronted by Venezuelan Christians, emphasizing the use of Venezuelan rhythms and instruments (Sifontes 2020). To demonstrate the concept, the network produced a crowdsourced a version of the well-known Latin American worship song, *Cuán bello es el Señor* (How beautiful the Lord) (AeC 2020c), which was quickly released on 7 April of 2020, scarcely 15 days after lockdowns had started in many countries, including Venezuela. The arrangement of the song was done using *Onda Nueva*, a Venezuelan musical style that fuses Venezuelan *joropo* with jazz and bossanova; sixteen worship leaders, singers, and musicians joined the project.

A multi-track model for the virtual ensemble was used, in which individual members recorded their part and a coordinator assemble the different pieces into a complete recording or video (Daffern et al. 2021). Although conceptually simple, the implementation required several steps to follow that depended on the technology available. Daffern et al. (2021) distinguish the role of the facilitator and of the participant in the recording. In the case of AeC, the facilitator, Ronald Sifontes, had a lot of experience editing audio and video, as well as the musical ability to create the backing tracks for the rest of the participants. Due to the lockdown, the equipment used was minimal, without access to the studio and other sophisticated audio interfaces. Moreover, uploading and downloading audio/video files was done using mobile broadband, which in the city of Merida is rather unstable and with a low throughput[4]. Additionally, the facilitator of AeC had to coordinate with participants their different contributions, organize the received recordings, edit them into a final product, uploading it to the social media sites, or distributing it via WhatsApp or Telegram. Participating members had to learn the new songs, create a minimal set-up to record their solo track, following the pre-recorded backing track created by the facilitator. The majority of AeC members used their mobile phones as recording device, having to make their recordings when their houses were quiet, many times in closets or bathrooms, or late at night, taking into consideration that everybody was staying home. Due to the peculiarities of life in Venezuela, a country without gasoline, with daily electricity outages, and an obsolete telecommunications infrastructure, worsened by the pandemic, all the musical production work faced big challenges. As members of the network described it:

> After videos were published, we asked ourselves, how did we do this? We did it by the grace and mercy of God. Without recording studio, many hours of patient editing with simple software tools, working around electricity cuts that did not have fixed schedules, sometimes working the night shifts until daybreak, using old computers, outdated smartphones, recording in crowded houses because of the lockdowns. (a member of AeC)

The precarious situation faced in Venezuela, exacerbated by the new living restrictions imposed by the lockdowns, created a sense of social instability or disequilibrium, a disruption from normal life, something that could be classified as a *liminal* state. According to Victor Turner, precisely in *liminality*, when things are confused and risks abound, is where a transient society, a *communitas*, emerges spontaneously, to undertake the goal of collective transformation (Turner 1969). Liminal states, such as the one produced by the pandemic, are characterized by their transient nature, humility, unselfishness, simplicity, suffering, spiritual growth, absence of rank and status, solidarity, togetherness, all of which facilitate the emergence of a *communitas*. AeC became a *communitas* formed around worship musicking, that provided a safe space for co-creation, imaginative engagement, redefining personal mission, experimentation, and learning together. Early members of AeC felt that something needed to be done despite the limitations, as one of the would put it: "We know that excellent equipment and instruments are necessary, but if we don't have them then, are we not going to do what we should?" (VyV 2020).

By reflecting on the encounters of the disciples with Jesus in John 20, a project to crowdsource the composition of original songs was started in the early months of the pandemic. Two original songs, *Tú Vives* (You are alive) (AeC 2020a) and *Sopla tu aliento en mi* (Blow your breath on me) (AeC 2020d), were the network's products of this challenge. In *Túl Vives*, using a modernized *gaita* rhythm from Zulia (Venezuela) state, a saddened Mary Magdalene returns to the tomb of Jesus. Her pain increases when she sees that the body of Jesus had disappeared. However, Jesus, calling her by name, reveals that he is alive. With a joyful heart she adores him and runs to announce the miracle to the other disciples. The song was intended to minister to the health workers caring for those suffering the complications of the viral infection, who were seeing so much death, but who were also meeting Jesus in many new ways. The song invites them to adore him, and to receive renewed strength to continue with their mission. *Sopla tu aliento en mi* enacts the breathing of Jesus on his disciples, sending them to fulfill the Great Commission (John 20:22–23). The song has an arrangement that mixes Venezuelan Caribbean rhythms of *gaita tamborera* (another musical genre of Zulia state) and *sangueo* (a drum-based rhythm from Aragua state in the central coast). People located in different countries contributed with the lyrics, playing instruments, singing, and in producing the Youtube WMV. One of the singers, a professional musician working for a dance orchestra in Spain, was so struck by the song that he decided to collaborate. Among the contributors to both lyrics and music, were California Vineyard pastors, Daniel and Nicole Hernández, for whom the rhythmic proposal that resulted, invited the incorporation of body movements to give glory to the Lord, in a way that facilitates an encounter with God that is truly Latin American.

At some point on the evolution of AeC, the themes for composition shifted to intercessory/prophetic lyrics. Several songs were produced putting emphasis on a vision of the rebuilding of the country. One of them, *Gloria al Todopoderoso (Glory to the Almighty)*

(AeC 2021) has a melody that can be classified as an anthem due to its rhythm and style. It is a song that seeks to honor God and expresses gratefulness for the immense riches which he granted to Venezuela. This song has been well received among Venezuelan Christians, especially in diasporic communities. Ronald Sifontes, who wrote and produced the contemporary anthem, says:

> For several months I had the phrases *Gloria al Todopoderoso* (glory to the Almighty) and *tierra de gracia y paz*[5] (land of grace and peace), but it was not until September (2020), when I was able to finish composing the song. The song declares gratitude for all the goodness that God has given us, like the beautiful geography and richness of our land, and the beauty of our big-hearted people. The stanzas are a compendium of statements of faith that describe the Venezuela we want to enjoy and see prosper. The music has that traditional air of a hymn, with melodic intervals that evoke hope, joy, strength, and peace. (Entrecristianos 2021)

The entire AeC network, and many more people who were recruited, participated with their voices, giving a choral sound, filled with energy, enthusiasm, and conviction. The song has been featured in many radio stations in state capitals and small towns all over the country, and it is played after the governmentally mandated Venezuelan anthem, *Gloria al bravo pueblo,* at designated times during the day. It has also been featured in recent *Marchas para Jesus* (March for Jesus) in several cities across Venezuela. According to musicologist Wershin Montiel (Montiel 2021), its success is mainly due to its melodic line and harmonic cycle which is simple to "linger" in the mind of the believers, although he finds the arrangement not so attractive to younger generations of believers. Some pastors from different parts of the country refer toa certain "atmosphere of grace" that the song creates, or of "the deep desire to see the nation restored and free from all oppressive yoke" declared by the lyrics, or even consider it as the "new national anthem". In this regard, a well known Pentecostal prophet from the Venezuelan Evangelical diaspora, envisions through the song the ideal of a new nation, of a country restored and rebuilt, with the just governance of God over the nation so that the chains of oppression are broken, yokes fall, and truth and light reign:

> This anthem was born from the heart of God. It expresses what many of us have believed through prophetic words. God is going to give us a new homeland. The old Venezuela is going to die to give rise to a new Venezuela. This is a proposal for an anthem for a new nation. In this hymn the glory is given to the God of heaven for being the creator and liberator of the new Venezuela. (Jose Hernandez, *Gethsemane Missionary Church*, Elkhart-Indiana, IN, USA)

In a similar fashion, the most popular of the AeC songs in Youtube, *Sana a Venezuela (Heal Venezuela)* (AeC 2020b), evokes the text of 2 Chronicles 7:14 and contextualizes its message to the situation of Venezuela with an oppressive regime and in a pandemic situation. The song is reminiscent of African American spirituals and some Psalms crying out to God in the midst of need and oppression. With a more Caribbean ballad rhythm, the center of the message focuses on the importance of turning to God with repentance about the mistakes made by earlier generations of Venezuelans, and to wait for God's intervention. This is also aligned with the widespread spiritual warfare teaching of *identificational repentance* (Holvast 2009). In this teaching, national collective iniquities give power to the forces of evil to dominate a territory or a nation, causing poverty, sickness, death, disasters, social disarray, which can be transmitted from one generation to the next. By identifying and confessing these collective sins, especially idolatry and immorality, current and future generations can be released of the consequences of the sin of their ancestors and from the demonic strongholds. Taking a more critical stance, Wershin Montiel points out that despite the beauty of the song, it promotes passivity among Christians because it transmits the belief that "only God can" deliver the country from a social disaster where the forces of evil had taken root, without other actions besides prayer and intercession (Montiel 2021).

5. Discussion

To conclude this paper, we revisit Heidi Campbell's framework introduced before (Campbell 2005), to analyze how AeC members perceive God's work in and through social networks, messaging applications, and the web in general (Sheldon and Campbell 2021). The main points of this framework are developed in relation to AeC as follows:

(1) *AeC was formed as a spiritual network* that sought to facilitate religious experience among Venezuelan Evangelical diasporic communities spread all over the world. The network was started once the lockdowns were initiated in most countries in the Americas. Over 50% of all AeC members belong to the Venezuelan Evangelical diaspora spread chiefly in South America, with additional members in the USA, Canada, Mexico, Costa Rica, and Spain. Besides, the musical aspect of the network, it serves as connection space where prayer support is provided, devotionals prepared by the members are shared, and religious news are distributed. For example, it was interesting see how AeC was invited to lead 24/7 warfare worship sessions as part of the national intercessory prayer movement during the week of 24 June of 2021, when several popular animist religious groups had been convened to do a commemorative ritual. AeC members viewed their network's participation as inspired by God.

(2) *AeC became a sacramental space for worship musicking.* Members of the network believed that God could be found in the possibility of interaction, the gracious listening of each other, the anointing to compose, and in how God touched those that watched their youtube WMV's or listened their recordings in WhatsApp. The pandemic provided an environment for co-writing worship music and lyrics where the usual pressures of offering a congregational worship set every Sunday, or the desire to please the Christian musical industry, were not present or at least were attenuated. As Dave Thornton has said, "creative collaboration is clearly most fertile in open environments of both benevolent honesty and goodwill" (Thornton 2021). AeC became a liminal *communitas* of vulnerable creative people who were not thinking on their own success and benefits, but who felt the need to contribute to the wellbeing of Venezuelan Christians wherever they may be.

(3) *AeC served to spread ideological and theological principles*, as well as religious practices. The desire of seeing God's intervention in the situation of Venezuela as a broken nation was present in almost all the compositions done by AeC. A *soft dominion theology* (Heuser 2021) is found in some of the songs, which comes from the widespread influence of the New Apostolic Reformation in the churches of the region, to which several of the members of AeC belong to. However, many times the common dichotomy between premillennial or postmillennial thought is present. Some songs describe a future where Venezuela is seen as a healed nation by God, where the kingdom of God can be realized. Others demonstrate a more escapist attitude of waiting passively for the rapture. Only the song *Sopla tu aliento en mi* calls for a more proactive missional impulse. None of the songs make explicit declarations on behalf of the poor, marginalized, or to denounce the injustice of Venezuelan society. The definition of sin and the appeal to purity, as understood by Evangelicals in Latin America, are also present in some of the compositions.

(4) *AeC successfully demonstrated the use of social media and technology to affirm and strengthen religious identity and community.* By the response of the Venezuelan diaspora to the songs it is possible to see that AeC came at a moment of great need due to the pandemic, but it also demonstrated that Venezuelan Evangelical migrants needed some reference to their faith from the homeland. Many of the members of AeC view this experience as a blessing of God confirmed by prophecy, but also as a miracle, if the extraordinary economic and technical limitations of Venezuelan society are taken into consideration. As a result, those congregated in the AeC network considered themselves as digital missionaries and worshippers for whom the Internet became a vehicle for God's work and mission.

We have attempted in this article to document how the network AeC emerged from the liminal state created by the pandemic, becoming a *communitas* seeking to contribute to churches and believers in a time of national and international struggle, disarray, and pain. The aim was to research AeC as unique case study in order to contribute to the fields of diaspora studies and religion, digital religion, new religious expressions, and lived religion during the pandemic. From this research several directions for more theoretical work can be identified such as the areas of Latin American contemporary worship music, the understanding of the sacramentality of digital worship, and the formation of new religious networks among migrants in Latin America, considering the current waves of Venezuelan, Cubans, Haitians, and Central Americans that traverse the continent in search of a "promise land" where they can flourish and fructify.

Author Contributions: F.A.M. was responsible of the conceptualization of the article. E.G.M. did all data collection, lead the focus group, and analysis. The two authors worked in the writing of the case study and the discussion. All authors have read and agreed to the published version of the manuscript.

Funding: This research received no external funding.

Acknowledgments: The authors are grateful to the AeC mebers that participated in the focus group despite the difficulty of distance and time differences. Also, we are indebted to Wershin Montiel in Santo Domingo, Dominican Republic, for his comments and Christian music analysis.

Conflicts of Interest: The authors declare no conflict of interest.

Notes

1 Versions from Australia, Burma, Chile, Canada, France, Ghana, India, Indonesia, Ireland, Italy, Lebanon, Madagascar, Malaysia, Mexico, the Netherlands, Nigeria, Romania, Spain, Singapore, South Africa, South Korea, Sweden, Vietnam, Zimbabwe, and an ensemble from Arab-speaking countries in the Middle East, North Africa, the Arabian Peninsula, Egypt, and South Sudan.

2 The designation *evangélicos* in Latin America encompass all Protestant expressions of Christianity. However, according to the cited PRC study, and many others, the majority of *evangélicos* are Pentecostal or Charismatic, although the latter term tends to not be used in order not to confuse with Catholic Charismatic Renewal. In this article, we use Evangelical in the Latin American sense, and, in most cases, we will be referring to Pentecostal Evangelicals.

3 The autor analyzed 26 songs from different artists and countries, all of them Latin American. The sample included well know artists such as Jorge Drexler, Juanes, Maná, Calle 13, Ricardo Arjona, Molotov, and Daddy Yankee, and different styles such as cumbia, reggaeton, reggae, pop, hip-hop, rap, rock, and trova.

4 Anecdotically speaking, to have better coverage for uploading or downloading music and videos, Ronald had to go out of his apartment searching for better signal power. In one of those instances, he got his cell phone stolen by a coupled of armed gang members.

5 It is important to remember that the first name of Venezuela, when Columbus hit the coast in his third trip to the Indies, was *Tierra de Gracia*. Later on, when the expedition reached Maracaibo Lake and saw the houses on the water, Americo Vespucio, called that Veznezuela which means "little Venice". That was the name that the Spanish crown ended up giving to the new possession.

References

Addo, Giuseppina. 2021. Join the Holy Spirit on Zoom: African Pentecostal churches and their liturgical practices during COVID-19. *Approaching Religion* 11: 45–61. [CrossRef]

AeC. 2020a. Available online: https://www.youtube.com/watch?v=noyxJhMkiMg (accessed on 27 November 2021).

AeC. 2020b. Available online: https://www.youtube.com/watch?v=R74taMbtx8E (accessed on 27 November 2021).

AeC. 2020c. Available online: https://www.youtube.com/watch?v=vVE4DRr8aTM (accessed on 27 November 2021).

AeC. 2020d. Available online: https://www.youtube.com/watch?v=Y1MmbW1Au1I (accessed on 27 November 2021).

AeC. 2021. Available online: https://www.youtube.com/watch?v=NUEHyOrFGIY (accessed on 27 November 2021).

Alonso, Andoni, and Pedro Oiarzabal. 2010. The Immigrant World's Digital Harbors: An Introduction. In *Diasporas in the New Media Age*. Edited by Andoni Alonso and Pedro Oiarzabal. Reno: University of Nevada Press, pp. 1–15.

Baumann, Martin. 2010. Exile. In *Diasporas: Concepts, Intersections, Identities*. Edited by Kim Knott and Sean McLoughlin. London: Zed Books, pp. 19–23.

Berhò, Deborah. 2020. An "Echo in the Soul": Worship Music in Evangelical Spanish-Language Latino Churches of Oregon. *Ecclesial Practices* 7: 203–25. [CrossRef]

Brueggemann, Walter. 1997. *Cadences of Home: Preaching among Exiles*. Louisville: Westminster John Knox Press.

Butler, Kim. 2001. Defining Diaspora, Refining a Discourse. *Diaspora: A Journal of Transnational Studies* 10: 189–219. [CrossRef]
Campbell, Heidi. 2005. Spiritualising the Internet. Uncovering Discourses and Narratives of Religious Internet Usage. *Heidelberg Journal of Religions on the Internet*. [CrossRef]
Campbell, Heidi, and Giulia Evolvi. 2020. Contextualizing current digital religion research on emerging technologies. *Human Behavior and Emerging Technologies* 2: 5–17. [CrossRef]
Campbell, Heidi, and Michael De Lashmutt. 2014. Studying Technology and Ecclesiology in Online Multi-Site Worship. *Journal of Contemporary Religion* 29: 267–85. [CrossRef]
Chaves-Gonzalez, Diego, and Carlos Echeverria-Estrada. 2020. *Venezuelan Migrants and Refugees in Latin American and the Caribbeas: A Regional Profile*. Washington, DC: Migration Policy Institute.
Chiu, Remi. 2020. Functions of Music Making under Lockdown: A Trans-Historical Perspective Across Two Pandemics. *Frontiers in Psychology* 11: 616499. [CrossRef]
Cunningham, Stuart, and David Craig. 2017. Being 'really real' on YouTube: Authenticity, community and brand culture in social media entertainment. *Media International Australia* 164: 71–81. [CrossRef]
Daffern, Helena, Kelly Balmer, and Jude Brereton. 2021. Singing Together, Yet Apart: The Experience of UK Choir Members and Facilitators during the COVID-19 Pandemic. *Frontiers in Psychology* 12: 624474. [CrossRef]
Entrecristianos. 2021. «Gloria al Todopoderoso» Claman Adoradores Venezolanos. *Entrecristianos*, October 7. Available online: https://bit.ly/36Ve8a9 (accessed on 27 November 2021).
Fowler, Megan. 2020. 'The Blessing' Sung Around the World:100 Virtual Choirs Spread Worship Anthem. *Christianity Today*, July 29.
Galdos, Guillermo, and Gena Somra. 2020. From Desperate for work, these immigrants collect the bodies of COVID-19 victims in Peru. *CNN*, October 5. Available online: https://cnn.it/2WFxY4e (accessed on 27 November 2021).
García Ayala, Daniela. 2019. Estrategias y Actitudes de Aculturación de un Grupo de Migrantes Venezolanos en Ecuador. Tesis de grado, Pontificia Universidad Católica de Ecuador, Ambato, Ecuador.
Gladwin, Ryan. 2015. Charismatic Music and the Pentecostalization of Latin American Evangelicalism. In *Spirit of Praise: Music and Worship in Global Pentecostal-Charismatic Christianity*. Edited by Monique Ingalls and Amos Yong. University Park: Penn State University Press, pp. 199–214.
Hansen, Niels, John Treider, Dana Swarbrick, Joshua Bamford, Johanna Wilson, and Jona Vuoskoski. 2021. Crowd-Sourced Database of Coronamusic: Documenting Online Making and Sharing of Music During the COVID-19 Pandemic. *Frontiers in Psychology* 12: 684083. [CrossRef]
Helland, Cristopher. 2016. Digital Religion. In *Handbook of Religion and Society*. Edited by David Yamane. Heidelberg: Springer, pp. 177–96.
Heuser, Andreas. 2021. Outlines of a Pentecostal Dominion Theology. In *Political Pentecostalism: Four Synoptic Surveys from Africa, Asia, and Latin America*. Edited by Leandro Fontana and Markus Luber. Frankfurt: Verlag Friederich Pustet, vols. 187–246.
Holvast, Rene. 2009. *Spiritual Mapping in the United States and Argentina 1989–2005: A Geography of Fear*. Leiden: Brill.
Ingalls, Monique. 2016. Worship on the Web: Broadcasting Devotion Through Worship Music Videos on YouTube. In *Music and the Broadcast Experience: Performance, Production, and Audiences*. Edited by Christina Baade and James Deaville. New York: Oxford University Press, pp. 293–308.
Instituto Nacional de Estadística de Venezuela. 2011. *Censo de Población y Vivienda de Venezuela 2011*. Caracas: INE.
Levitt, Peggy. 2007. Rezar por encima de las fronteras: Cómo los inmigrantes están cambiando el panorama religioso. *Migración y Desarrollo* 8: 66–86. [CrossRef]
Lim, Swee Hong, and Lester Ruth. 2017. *Lovin' on Jesus: A Concise History of Contemporary Worship*. Nashville: Abingdon Press.
Lupton, Donna, and Karen Willis. 2021. COVID Society. In *The COVID-19 Crisis: Social Perspectives*. Edited by Donna Lupton and Karen Willis. London: Routledge, pp. 3–13.
Mazzoli, Mattia, Boris Diechtiareff, Antónia Tugores, William Wives, Natalia Adler, Pere Colet, and Jose Ramasco. 2020. Migrant Mobility Flows Characterized With Digital Data. *PLoS ONE* 15: e0230264. [CrossRef] [PubMed]
McGarry, Patsy. 2020. Over 300 church groups unite for online Irish Blessing video. *The Irish Times*, May 31.
Meher, Mattias. 2022. WhatsApp, WeChat and Facebook Messenger Apps—Global Useage of Messaging Apps, Penetration and Statistics. Available online: https://bit.ly/2XmSg2u (accessed on 27 November 2021).
Montiel, Wershin. 2021. Independent Consultant in Music, Santo Domingo, Dominican Republic. Personal communication.
Onderdijk, Kelsy, Freya Acar, and Edith Van Dick. 2021. Impact of Lockdown Measures on Joint Music Making: Playing Online and Physically Together. *Frontiers in Psychology* 12: 642713. [CrossRef] [PubMed]
Pang, Natalie, and Yue Woo. 2020. What about WhatsApp? A systematic review of WhatsApp and its Role in Civic and Political Engagement. *First Monday* 25. [CrossRef]
Paniagua-Arguedas, Laura. 2017. Voces en Movimiento: Latinoamérica migrante dibujada por la música. *Revista Colombiana de Ciencias Sociales* 8: 479–501. [CrossRef]
Pérez Guadalupe, José. 2020. Brasil e os Novos Atores Religiosos da Política Latino-americana. In *Novo Ativismo Político no Brasil: Os Evangélicos do Século XXI*. Edited by José Luis Pérez Guadalupe and Brenda Carranza. Rio de Janeiro: Konrad Adenauer Stiftung, pp. 17–109.
Pérez, Adam. 2021. 'All Hail King Jesus': The International Worship Symposium and the Making of Praise and Worship History, 1977–1989. Ph.D. dissertation, Duke University, Durham, NC, USA.

Ponzanesi, Sandra. 2020. Digital Diasporas: Postcoloniality, Media and Affect. *Interventions: International Journal of Postcolonial Studies* 22: 977–93. [CrossRef]

PRC. 2014. *Religion in Latin America: Widespread Change in a Historically Catholic Region*. Washington, DC: Pew Research Center.

PRC. 2019. *Mobile Connectivity in Emerging Economies*. Washington, DC: Pew Research Center.

R4V: Plataforma Regional de Coordinación Interagencial. 2021. *Refugiados y Migrantes de Venezuela*. Available online: https://www.r4v.info/es/refugiadosymigrantes (accessed on 27 November 2021).

Roberts, Stephen. 2021. Listening to lockdown: Sound theology in a time of crisis. *Practical Theology* 14: 71–85. [CrossRef]

Rocha, Cristina. 2017. "The Come to Brazil Effect": Young Brazilians' Fascination with Hillsong. In *The Hillsong Movement Examined: You Call Me out upon the Waters*. Edited by Tanya Riches and Tim Wagner. Cham: Palgrave McMillan.

Rosenbusch, Hannes, Anthony Evans, and Marcel Zeelenberg. 2019. Multilevel Emotion Transfer on YouTube: Disentangling the Effects of Emotional Contagion and Homophily on Video Audiences. *Social Psychological and Personality Science* 10: 1028–35. [CrossRef]

Sabar, Galia, and Shlomit Kanari. 2006. 'I'm Singing my Way Up': The Significance of Music Amongst African Christian Migrants in Israel. *Studies in World Christianity* 12: 101–25.

Santos, Miguel Angel. 2018. ¿Cuántos son y qué Perfil Tienen los Venezolanos en el Exilio? Una Aproximación a Través de Facebook. Prodavinci. Available online: https://bit.ly/3hzTij0 (accessed on 27 November 2021).

Sheldon, Zachary, and Heidi Campbell. 2021. Divine Revelation and Digital Religion. In *The Oxford Handbook of Divine Revelation*. Edited by Balázs Mezei, Francesca Aran Murphy and Keneth Oakes. Oxford Handbooks Online. [CrossRef]

Sifontes, Ronald. 2020. *¿Qué es Adorando en Casa?* Available online: https://bit.ly/3K4AMuR (accessed on 27 November 2021).

Sim, Jaeung, Daegon Cho, Youngdeok Hwang, and Rahul Telang. 2020. Virus Shook the Streaming Star: Estimating the COVID-19 Impact on Music Consumption. *Marketing Science*. [CrossRef]

Simons, Helen. 2009. *Case study Research in Practice*. London: SAGE.

Siuda, Piotr. 2021. Mapping Digital Religion: Exploring the Need for New Typologies. *Religions* 12: 373. [CrossRef]

Small, Christopher. 1999. Musicking—The meanings of performing and listening: A lecture. *Music Education Research* 1: 9–22. [CrossRef]

Snider Andrews, Emily. 2019. Exploring Evangelical Sacramentality: Modern Worship Music and the Possibility of Divine-Human Encounter. Ph.D. dissertation, Fuller Theological Seminary, Center for Advance Theological Studies, Pasadena, CA, USA.

Starman, Adrijana Biba. 2013. The case study as a type of qualitative research. *Journal of Contemporary Educational Studies/Sodobna Pedagogika* 64: 28–43.

Thornton, Daniel. 2021. *Meaning-Making in the Contemporary Congregational Song Genre*. Cham: Palgrave McMillan.

Turner, Victor. 1969. Liminality and Communitas. In *The Ritual Process: Structure and Anti-Structure*. Edited by Victor Turner. Chicago: Aldine Publishing, pp. 94–113.

Vásquez, Manuel. 2008. Studying Religion in Motion: A network approach. *Method and Theory in the Study of Religion* 20: 151–84. [CrossRef]

Vélez Caro, Constanza, and Miguel Mansilla. 2019. Espacios Sonoros: La Música como Recurso Simbólico en los Migrantes Peruanos y Bolivianos Pentecostales de la Ciudad de Iquique. *Sociedad y Religión* 34: 12–39.

VyV. 2020. Adorando en Casa: Música Venezolana para Dios. *Verdad y Vida*, September 30. Available online: https://bit.ly/3od5DxK (accessed on 27 November 2021).

MDPI AG
Grosspeteranlage 5
4052 Basel
Switzerland
Tel.: +41 61 683 77 34

Religions Editorial Office
E-mail: religions@mdpi.com
www.mdpi.com/journal/religions

www.ingramcontent.com/pod-product-compliance
Lightning Source LLC
Chambersburg PA
CBHW062106220926
51850CB00010B/2909